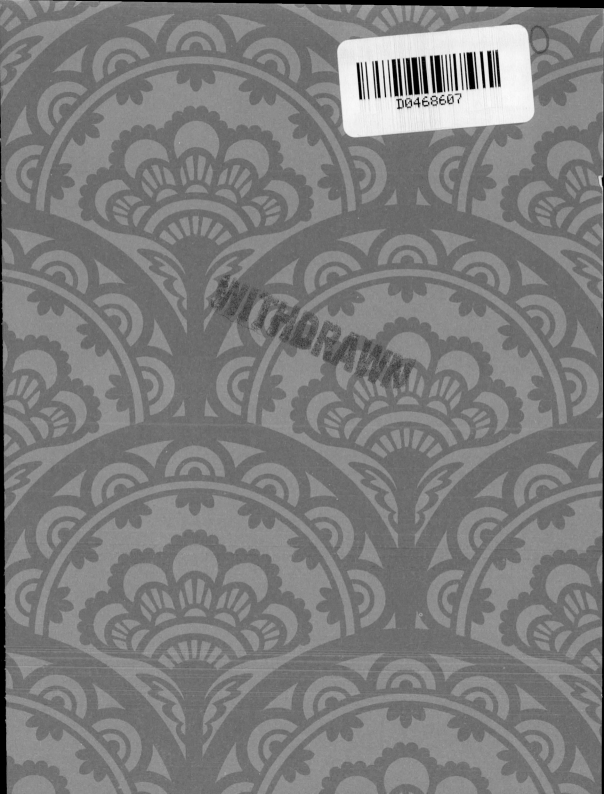

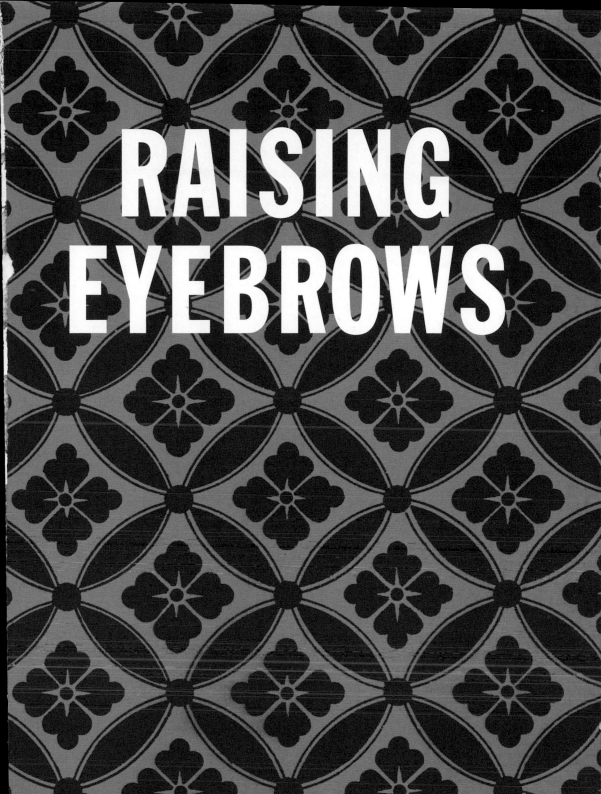

RAISING
EYEBROWS

RAISING
EYEBROWS

*your personal guide
to fabulous brows*

BY CAMERON TUTTLE

CHRONICLE BOOKS

SAN FRANCISCO

PUBLISHED EXCLUSIVELY FOR BENEFIT COSMETICS BY CHRONICLE BOOKS LLC.

Text copyright © 2011 by Benefit Cosmetics LLC
Illustrations copyright © 2011 by Anne Keenan Higgins/Illo Reps, Inc.

Photographs copyright © 2011 by Christopher Kern with the exception of photographs on the following pages: 12 (©iStockphoto.com/Knape); 32 Nefertiti (AP Photo/ Markus Schreiber, File), cosmetics box (Gianni Dagli Orti / Photolibrary); 36 (©iStockphoto.com/Mikhail Khromov); 38 (Queen Elizabeth I by Marcus Gheeraerts, the Younger (c.1561-1635) (after) Wimpole Hall, Cambridgeshire, UK/National Trust Photographic Library/Christopher Hurst/Bridgeman Art Library); 45 Dietrich (AP Photo), Kahlo (Detroit Institute of Arts, USA/ The Bridgeman Art Library); 46 Taylor (AP Photo), Twiggy (AP Photo); 48 (AP Photo/Kathy Willens); 50 Carter (AP Photo), Ann-Margret (AP Photo); 51 Brando (AP Photo), Gable (NBCU Photo Bank via AP Images); 56 Diaz (Evan Agostini/ PictureGroup via AP Images), Beyonce (AP Photo/Jim Cooper), Moore (AP Photo/Danny Moloshok), Witherspoon (AP Photo/Kevork Djansezian, File); 69 (©iStockphoto.com/Drazen Vukelic); 107 (AP Photo/Jorge Herrera, File).

ISBN: 978-1-4521-1133-9

Library of Congress Cataloging-in-Publication data is available.

Manufactured in China.

Design by Tracy Sunrize Johnson.
Hair and makeup by Alex LaMarsh and assistant Rebecca Butz.
Brows by Hilary Foote.

Accutane is a trademark of the F. Hoffman-La Roche Ltd.; Band-Aid is a registered trademark of Johnson & Johnson Consumer Companies, Inc.; Benefit is a registered trademark of Benefit Cosmetics LLC; Benefit BrowBar is a registered trademark of Benefit Cosmetics LLC; Botox is a registered trademark of Allergan, Inc.; BrowBar is a registered trademark of Benefit Cosmetics LLC; Differin is a registered trademark of Galderma Laboratories, L.P.; Renova is a registered trademark of Ortho, a division of Ortho-McNeil-Janssen Pharmaceuticals, Inc.; Retin-A is a registered trademark of OrthoNeutrogena; Tri-Luma is a registered trademark of Galderma Laboratories, L.P.; Tweezerman is a registered trademark of Tweezerman International, Inc.

10 9 8 7 6 5 4 3 2 1

Chronicle Books LLC
680 Second Street
San Francisco, California 94107

www.chroniclebooks.com/custom

Contents

INTRODUC

YOU NEVER KNOW WHEN YOUR NEXT BROW-RAISING, LIFE-CHANGING OPPORTUNITY WILL PRESENT ITSELF.

There I was, getting my eyebrows shaped at my local Benefit Brow Bar in San Francisco, when my fave brow babe asked what book I would be writing next. I smiled sweetly, pretending to contemplate her question while I cringed inside and tried to ignore the panicked voice in my head, *Next book? Next BOOK? I have no idea!*

At certain *uncertain* times, asking a writer about her next book is a lot like asking, "How much more weight do you hope to lose?" or, "Still Internet dating?"

Before I could answer and sputter some painful, embarrassing truth, she saved me. "Hey, why don't you write a book about eyebrows? They're incredibly, amazingly fascinating."

I laughed.

Was she kidding? I mean, seriously. Who could write an entire book about *eyebrows*?!

Apparently me.

When I sat down to research and write this book, I hadn't given eyebrows much thought, other than wondering if mine made me look better or worse. But that brow babe was right. Eyebrows *are* incredibly, amazingly fascinating!

TION

Turns out they're not only an object of beauty with a rich, colorful past; they're also a personal power tool for better verbal and nonverbal communication and *the* most important feature in facial recognition. What does this mean? **EVERYONE IS LOOKING AT YOUR EYEBROWS.**

Now? Oh. My. God. Brows are my new best friend and my favorite new beauty habit rolled into one. Everywhere I go, I see brows—gorgeously groomed brows, neglected droopy brows, brows with personality, brows with a lot to say, strong brows, wispy brows, and wonderfully expressive wow brows.

I have learned that every brow is beautiful and unique and deserves to be loved—and that every brow has a story. Hmm. Maybe my next book will be an eyebrow memoir. But I digress. If you've ever doubted the importance of your eyebrows or thought that good brow behavior was beneath you (or beyond you!), your brow world is about to be rocked. A great brow shaping can make you look younger, thinner, happier, and richer. Seriously. It's like an instant face-lift!

I hope you enjoy this adventure through the past, present, and future of fabulous eyebrows as much as I enjoyed writing it! And please, always put your best brow forward. You never know when that next life-changing opportunity will present itself—an old boyfriend on the street, a new business opportunity at a party, your blog post goes viral—leading to a multiple book deal and a TV show based on **BEAUTIFUL YOU!**

1

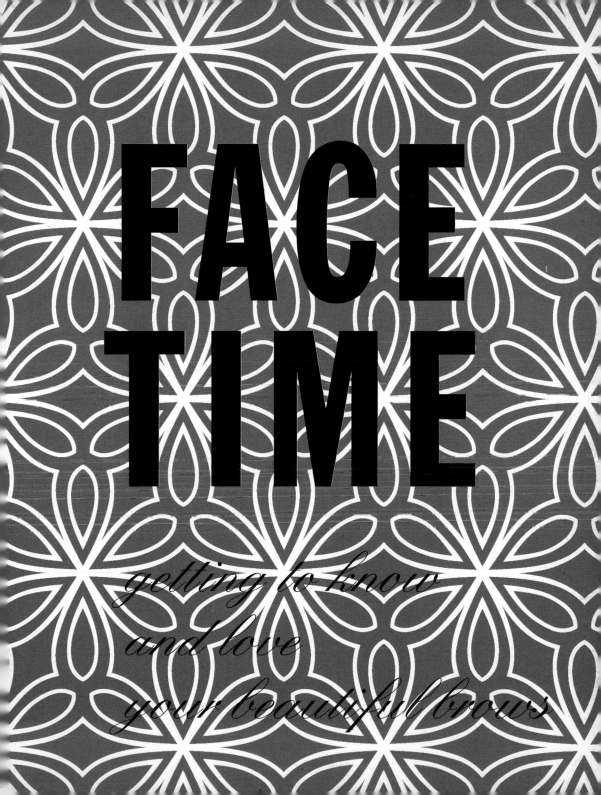

FACE TIME

getting to know and love your beautiful brows

RAISING EYEBROWS IS THE FEMININE POWER OF WOW!

It's the art of personal style that turns heads when you walk through an airport and draws attention when you enter a room. Raising eyebrows is communicating, it's connecting, it's flirting—it's fun. And it's the international language for *Hello, beautiful!*

**IN ANY LANGUAGE, A RAISED EYEBROW SAYS, I'M INTERESTED!
TWO RAISED EYEBROWS SAY, I'M INTERESTING—AWAKE, ALIVE, CURIOUS,
AND I'VE GOT IT GOING ON!**

Raising eyebrows is more than the ability to allure—it's proof that your allure is working. Seeing those eyebrows going up all around you is the ultimate compliment and zero-calorie immediate gratification.

Are you in? Want to know the secret to raising the eyebrows around you?

It all starts with raising your own brows.

Raising your eyebrows is a lot like raising children. All your brows need is love, support, and a little guidance to lead happy, healthy fulfilling lives—*and* to be there for you through thick and thin! But before you can raise your eyebrows to perfection, you have to know them.

WHEN DID YOU LAST spend quality alone time with your brows? Last month? Last year? Last never? Would you describe your relationship with your eyebrows as:

- *Barely there?*
- *Rough around the edges?*
- *All over the place?*

- *Disconnected?*
- *Too connected (aka codependent)?*
- *Happy and healthy?*

Do you really even know your brows? **?**

the time is
BROW!

Sadly, eyebrows are often the unloved and neglected stepchildren in the family of facial features. Why? Not because eyes and lips are better! They just demand more attention. The typical eyebrow is simply misunderstood. Most people—even the makeup savvy and the cosmetic queen—don't take the time to really get to know their brows and understand their needs. It's time to change all that. It's time for every man, woman, and child to accept that brows are real and that they need your love and attention.

WHAT ARE YOU WAITING FOR? Now is the time to get to know your brows, understand their needs, and show them some big love.

Grab a good mirror, sit down, and get comfortable. You're about to get up close and personal with your eyebrows and see them for what they really are—amazing!

function before fashion

The original purpose of the eyebrow was all function—to protect your eye from rain and sweat. If you take a close look at your own brows, you'll see a beautiful work of natural design. The overall arched shape of the brow works with the individual hairs— some growing straight up, some growing down, others growing sideways—to make a sleek, sexy little rain gutter. Cool, huh? So when a drop of moisture hits your eyebrow, your brow catches the drop and redirects the flow sideways around the eye.

the hidden power of the brow

Not only do your brows protect your eyes, but they're also highly trained communications specialists. Angry? Check the brows. Surprised? Check the brows. Worried? Check the brows. Attracted? Check the brows. Unlike other facial features that can easily deceive (sorry, mouth!), the eyebrows don't lie. Certain feelings, thoughts, and reactions set off a physical reflex that makes the eyebrows do their thing— move and communicate. Eyebrows are like punctuation marks to your emotions. They help you communicate to others and understand what others are trying to communicate to you. What eyebrows say and how they say it is virtually universal, crossing gender, age, cultural, and socioeconomic boundaries. Who knew? Eyebrows are the universal language of deep emotion!

Now look in the mirror and see for yourself. Do some warm-up exercises to limber up—raise one brow, raise both brows, do a little eyebrow dance. Now see what your brows do when you send a few nonverbal messages to yourself.

I'M TERRIFIED!

I'M SURPRISED!

I MUST KISS YOU NOW!

Can you match your facial expressions with these thoughts and feelings? Of course you can! The brows say it all.

Eyebrows don't just punctuate the big emotions; they also work hard to suggest very subtle, nonverbal social cues, especially to the opposite sex.

WHAT YOUR EYEBROWS CAN SAY

without a word

- I'm interested. Tell me more.
- I feel your pain.
- I don't believe a word you're saying.
- I'm bored.
- I'm flirting with intent.
- Oh my God. No way!
- Please get over here and offer to buy me a drink.

Eyebrows also play a key role in face recognition. According to recent research in the development of artificial face-recognition systems, eyebrows actually play a more important role in face recognition than eyes. When participants looked at the photos of well-known actors and politicians, they were far less able to identify the person when the *eyebrows* were removed from the photos than they were when the eyes were removed.

Even the experts didn't see that one coming.

RESEARCH CONCLUSION: Eyebrows are more important than eyes in helping you recognize someone.

LIFE CONCLUSION: Even if *you* aren't focusing on your eyebrows, everyone else is!

Eyebrows also help us identify gender, especially from a distance. This is not just based on social conditioning or fashion; it's in our DNA. Eyebrow researchers have concluded that humans are genetically coded to associate brow thickness with gender. A thick, bushy brow says *strong man* to us, somewhere deep in the brain. A light or wispy brow says *young boy* or *woman*. Eyebrows give us a quick cue to tell the men from the boys and the men from the women, whether it's across the wide-open plains or a crowded dance floor.

*

NOTE TO BROW:
LET'S NOT BE MISTAKEN FOR A DUDE.

WE CAN ACTUALLY SEE THE EVIDENCE OF HUMAN EVOLUTION in the development of the eyebrow. In prehistoric times, brows were prominent and fixed (think caveman). Not much subtle communication was required when running for your life from dinosaurs or woolly mammoths. By comparison, today our eyebrows are fine-tuned instruments of expression that can move together, move independently, and even do some crazy caterpillar dancing.

WITHOUT EYEBROWS, THE WORLD WOULD BE A SCARY PLACE. No one would recognize anyone or understand what anyone was saying! Fortunately, our eyebrows are here to stay.

Brow-Raising facts

● In sign language—the ultimate form of nonverbal communication—eyebrow movements indicate the difference between a statement and a question. The eyebrows also help suggest skepticism, irony, and doubt.

● The average cost of a brow-lift performed by a cosmetic surgeon is around $2,500. The average cost of a brow shaping performed by a cosmetic professional is about $25.*

* THE ADDED BENEFIT

At a Benefit Brow Bar or Boutique, a highly trained expert with fresh breath and a great personality will shape your brows to perfection for less than $25. And you don't even need an appointment! Full-frontal disclosure: The brow experts at Benefit are the beauty *and* the brains behind this book.

● Complete eyebrow loss can occur in both men and women. It's most commonly caused by injury, trauma, overplucking, or aging. Yikes! (In the United States, more than 3 million people lose their eyebrows every year.)

● Wigs for eyebrows? **YES!** Eyebrow wigs are made from human hair woven into a delicate lace base and then stuck to the skin with an adhesive.

● Camels have three eyebrows—one above each eye and one large tufted crest in the middle. Why? To protect the eyes from harsh sun and blowing sand.

● A New York salon now offers eyebrow hair extensions. Seriously. Individual strands of human hair are superglued to existing brow hairs and to the skin to extend and define the shape of the brow. Unfortunately, the extensions only last about two weeks.

what makes eyebrows unique?

Everything.

● *Eyebrow hairs grow individually, one per follicle.*
(The hair on your head grows in one to four hair follicular units.)

● *The average life span of the hairs that make up your eyebrow is just four months. (The typical scalp hair will live from three to seven years.)*

● *Eyebrows are the slowest growing hair on the body.*
(Thank goodness they start growing in at different times so they don't all have the same expiration date.)

● *A shaved brow can take up to a year to grow back completely.*
(Fortunately, most of it grows back in about two months.)

WHY *shape your brows?*

There are so many reasons—all of them good!

- It's what separates us from animals in the wild.
- It's a simple way to make a big difference in how you look.
- In many cultures, shaping the brows is a right of passage. (In other words, it's what real women do!)
- Everyone is always looking at your brows (even if you aren't)!

Well-shaped brows define your eyes and refine your whole look. They finish and polish your features. They refresh, brighten, and open your eyes. They can even make you look younger, thinner, and more refreshed. Great brow shaping is the ultimate instant face-lift!

Brows that are not groomed into the best shape for your face can really work against you. If your eyebrows are thick, they can make you look heavier than you are. If they're droopy and low, they can make you look tired. If they're thin and wispy, they can make you look washed-out and weak—and no one wants that!

Well-shaped eyebrows improve your look in so many ways. Shaping your brows to follow the best natural lines can take stress, years, and pounds off your face.

REALLY.

oh my brow!

The first time you have your eyebrows shaped and styled by a professional, don't be surprised if something like this comes out of your mouth:

"WOW. I LOOK TEN YEARS YOUNGER!"

"HELLO, GORGEOUS! WAIT . . . THAT'S ME?!"

"(GASP!) I JUST LOST FIVE POUNDS."

"IS IT JUST ME, OR DO I LOOK HAPPIER/NICER/FRIENDLIER/RICHER?"

"OMG! I LOOK SO GOOD, I'M ATTRACTED TO MYSELF!"

No matter what comes out of your mouth, you'll definitely look better with well-shaped brows. And don't worry. You won't look like someone else. You'll just look like you—the best you.

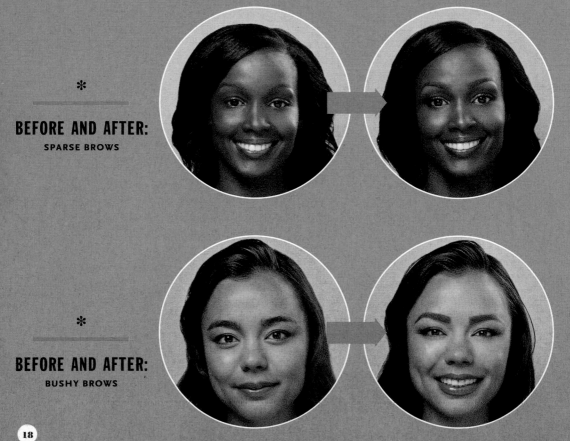

＊

BEFORE AND AFTER:
SPARSE BROWS

＊

BEFORE AND AFTER:
BUSHY BROWS

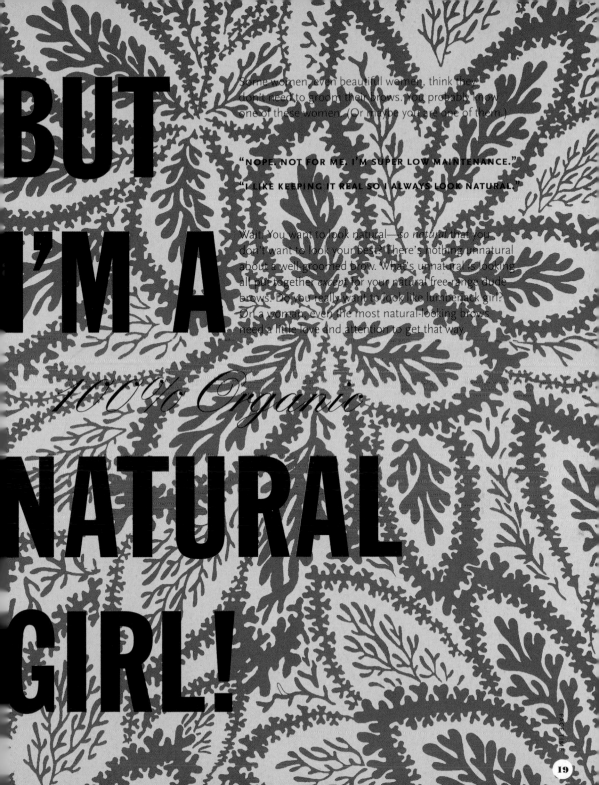

BUT I'M A NATURAL GIRL!

Some women, even beautiful women, think they don't need to groom their brows. You probably know one of these women. (Or maybe you are one of them.)

"NOPE, NOT FOR ME. I'M SUPER LOW MAINTENANCE."

"I LIKE KEEPING IT REAL SO I ALWAYS LOOK NATURAL."

Wait. You want to look natural—*so natural* that you don't want to look your best? There's nothing unnatural about a well-groomed brow. What's unnatural is looking all put together *except* for your natural, free-range dude brows. Do you really want to look like lumberjack girl? On a woman, even the most natural-looking brows need a little love and attention to get that way.

100% Organic

popular excuses for ignoring/neglecting your brows

There are plenty of reasons to neglect your eyebrows—but no *good* reasons. Okay, there is **ONE GOOD REASON.** Can you find it?

● *I'm super busy.*

● *I'm afraid that once I start tweezing, I won't be able to stop.*

● *I can't find them.*

● *I can't use my tweezers—they're my cat's new favorite toy!*

● *I'm not sure what to do.*

● *I'm not dating anyone.*

● *I'm waiting for the totally natural look that was never really in to come back.*

● *I'm Bohairhemian.*

● *I'm too young.*

● *I'm too old.*

● *Looking good is not in my budget.*

● *I believe that each and every hair is God's creation and deserves to live.*

● *None of my friends are doing it.*

● *Wait. Brows plural?*

If you answered *None of my friends are doing it*, you're wrong. Some of your friends are definitely doing it. Maybe even all your friends. A few might even be doing it together. But if you haven't noticed, then they're doing it well. They look foxy and fabulous, and the shape of their brows looks completely natural. That could be you!

If you guessed *I'm not sure what to do*, you're correct! That is the only good reason for neglecting your brows. Fortunately, you're holding this book, so that's all about to change.

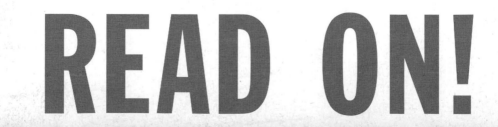

READ ON!

But wait!
I'M STILL WORRIED.

SOME TRUE AND FALSE QUESTIONS ABOUT BROW SHAPING

THE Q

1. Tweezing is a gateway habit to more serious stuff. True or false?

2. Any hair I remove will grow back darker, thicker, and faster than before. True or false?

3. If I shape my brows, I'll look constantly surprised. True or false?

4. If a hair falls in a brow forest and no one is there to . . . Hmm. Never mind.

THE A

1. *True!* Tweezing is a gateway habit to serious grooming and glamour!

2. *False.* The truth is, repeated removal of unwanted hairs sends a message to the individual hair follicles: "Honey, your services are no longer needed." Over time the follicle gets the message and goes on a permanent vacation. No more new hair!

3. *True!* You'll look constantly surprised by how much better and more refreshed you appear!

4. *No one knows.*

FACE TIME

21

are you more than just worried?

Do you ever experience eyebrow shame? Do you fear your brows without knowing why? If so, you could be suffering from **PTTD** (post-traumatic tweezing disorder).

Don't be afraid to admit it. It happens to the best, the brightest, the most beautiful. It might have happened in high school on a lonely Friday night or during college when someone very, very special went away for the weekend and didn't call, even though he'd said he would—in fact, he'd promised. Twice! It could have happened in your twenties with your roommates after too much wine and reality TV. Maybe it happened last month after that phone call with your mother. You tweezed your brows into oblivion or perhaps just into a very, very, very thin, high arch.

Whatever the circumstances, **IT'S OKAY.** You went tweezer crazy—it happens—and now you've got pain, shame, guilt, and fear associated with grooming your brows.

If you do suffer from PTTD, you also may be experiencing brow denial—neglecting them, ignoring them, pretending they don't even exist. Or perhaps you're still actively abusing your brows— feeling helpless and alone, trapped in the self-destructive vicious circle of overtweezing and unsure of how to break free! You can. And you will.

HEALTHY, HAPPY BROWS ARE ONLY A FEW PAGES AWAY.

Let's

LOOK IN THE MIRROR AGAIN
AND ASK A FEW TOUGH QUESTIONS.

1. Are your brows a crazy mess and completely out of control?
Look closely. Be honest. Are your brows terrorizing the rest of your face?
Oh no. Have you become . . . *Browzilla?*

2. Do your brows look like tiny little egg baskets?
Are you secretly trying to fulfill your nesting desires in your eyebrows?
Oh dear. Nesting. We all get the urge to do it at some point. We're women.
It's in our DNA, our TMI, our WTF. We nest. It's what we do.
But let's be clear: eyebrows are not for nesting.

3. Are your eyebrows drooping or sagging with no visible sign of support?
Do you have Cross-Your-Heart Brows—brows you promised to love
and support way back when but never got around to doing it?
It's not too late! Your brows can look perky again and make heads turn.
All they need is your loving support.

OR IS IT EVEN WORSE THAN THAT?

4. Have you been leaving the house *browless*? Grocery shopping browless
in front of your neighbors and their children? Going to work browless?
Jogging browless? Are you nuts?! It may not feel bad right now,
but you will definitely regret it later—when you see pictures. Of yourself.
Browless. Anywhere. Everywhere. Especially all over Facebook.

Whether you've got PTTD or you're just not sure
what to do with your brows, it's time to turn the page.
Take a quick tour of brow-shaping basics, the same principles
used by the pros (brow experts and licensed aestheticians),
and you'll see how easy it is to improve your brows—
and to give them the love and attention
they deserve.

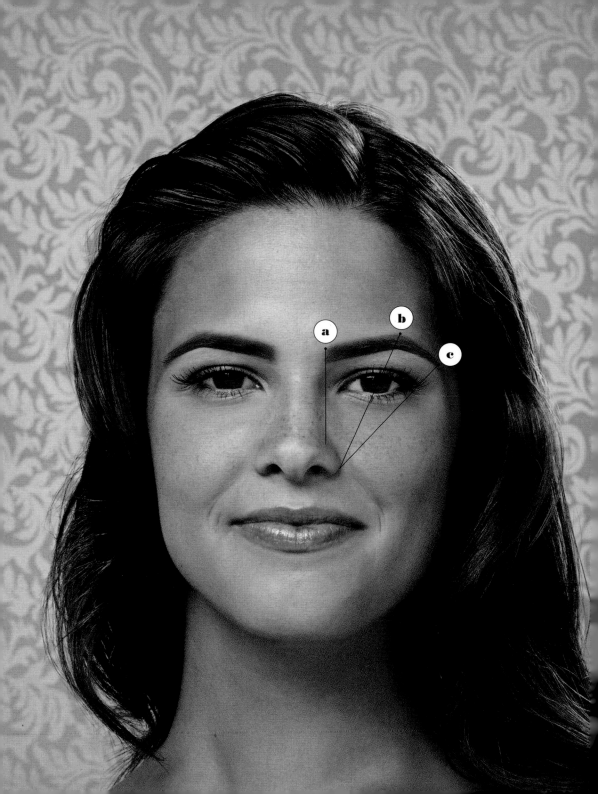

BROW-SHAPING *Basics*

(LOOK BUT DON'T TOUCH!)

Now let's get even closer to the mirror and learn the basic principles for shaping the eyebrow. If you're holding tweezers, drop them right now! Seriously. This is the *just browsing* section.

The basics for shaping your brow are as easy as **a b c**.

WHAT YOU NEED: A mirror you can get close to, plenty of natural light, and a pencil, chopstick, or any other thin, straight-edged object that's easy to hold and not too sharp.

Be sure to look straight ahead into that mirror during all this. (No Facebook profile shots, please!) You may look super alluring glancing up or to the side—but not now. Your brows need your undivided attention!

point a is the start of the brow.

point b is the highest point of the arch.

point c is the end of the brow.

FINDING YOUR NATURAL POINT A

WHAT YOU DO: Hold the pencil along the side of the bridge of your nose, resting it in the dimple where the nostril begins, with the pencil pointing straight up. Where that line extends to the eyebrow is your natural Point A, the best spot for your brow to start. Now try it yourself in the mirror.

WHAT DO YOU SEE? If the start of your brow is right on your natural Point A, then you don't need to change a thing. But if your brow starts beyond your natural Point A or doesn't quite extend enough to reach it, great news: You've got an opportunity for brow improvement!

FINDING YOUR NATURAL POINT B

WHAT YOU DO: Hold the pencil along the outside edge of your nostril, and then align it with the center of your pupil. Where that line extends to the eyebrow is your natural Point B, the highest point of your brow's arch. Now try it yourself in the mirror.

WHAT DO YOU SEE? If the highest point of your brow is right on your natural Point B, then you don't need to change a thing. But if it's off in either direction or not quite there at all, then it's time to show your brow some love and get it into better shape. Wait. Not yet! Put down those tweezers.

ARE YOU EXCEPTIONAL?

IF YOU HAVE EXCEPTIONALLY WIDE-SET EYES, EXCEPTIONALLY CLOSE-SET EYES, OR AN EXCEPTIONALLY BROAD NOSE, THEN YOU'LL WANT TO MODIFY THESE PRINCIPLES A BIT. SEE PAGE 59 FOR TIPS ON HOW TO USE YOUR BROW AS A SECRET BEAUTY WEAPON TO IMPROVE THE BALANCE OF YOUR FEATURES.

FINDING YOUR NATURAL POINT C

WHAT YOU DO: Hold the pencil along the outside edge of your nostril, and then align it with the outside edge of your eye. Where that line extends to the eyebrow is your natural Point C, the best place for your brow to end. Now try it yourself in the mirror.

WHAT DO YOU SEE? If the end of your brow comes to a graceful, defined point right on your natural Point C, then you're a miracle! That hardly ever occurs in nature. Chances are your end stops a little short of your best Point C *or* you've got a few stragglers (maybe lots) heading north or south on the temple trail. In either case, it's an easy fix, with eye-lifting results.

Remember, these are just the basics to get you excited about the shape of brows to come. In chapter 3, we'll go into more specifics to help you discover the best brow shape for you.

okay,

Personal Assessment Time

Take a deep breath and a good, long, up-close-and-personal look in the mirror. It's time to accept your brows for what they are and love them for what they can be—beautiful and uniquely you.

TAKE THE BROW EXAM!

PENCILS UP! Get up close to a mirror, be brave, and be honest.

1. Do you have any free-range hairs above or below the brow?

2. Do your brows start with a bang and end with a whimper?

3. Is your natural Point A *not* aligned with the start of your brow?

4. Do the inner corners of your brows look like tiny birds' nests?

5. Could a guy look good wearing your brows?

6. Do you have bald spots, thin patches, or female-pattern brow balding?

7. Is your natural Point B *not* aligned with the highest point of your brow arch?

8. When you look in the mirror and take ten paces back, do your brows disappear?

9. Do your brows hang low and need a lift?

10. Do they wobble to and fro and need a trim?

11. Are you wearing a Cross-Your-Heart Brow or going completely browless?

12. Is your natural Point C *not* aligned with the end of your brow?

13. Is one brow higher or lower than the other? Bigger or smaller? (It's okay. This is true for everyone!)

14. Is there anything you don't love about your brows?

PENCILS DOWN! If you answered yes to any of these questions, you've got an opportunity to get your brows in better shape so you can look your best. And as they say, opportunity rocks!

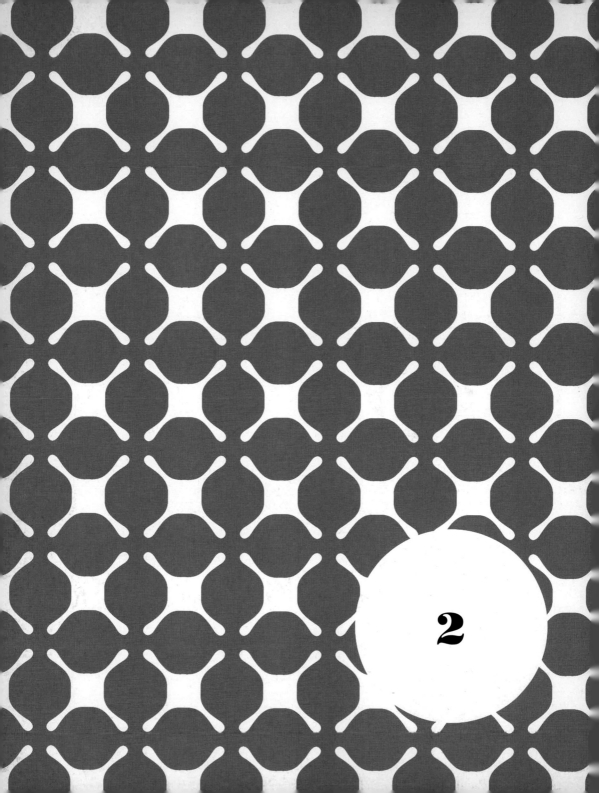

2

BROW HISTORY

ONE-OH-FUN!

the fascinating journey of the eyebrow through the ages

THE HISTORY OF THE EYEBROW AND OF EYE
ADORNMENT IS AS FASCINATING AS THE
STRONG AND STYLISH WOMEN WHO LIVED IT.
OKAY, SIT UP STRAIGHT FOR A MINUTE—
THIS IS SERIOUSLY COOL STUFF.

THANKS TO ARCHAEOLOGISTS, ARTISTS, AND THE POETS, novelists, and common
everyday journal-scribbling fanatics who left detailed notes through the ages, we
have a surprisingly good idea today of how eyebrow shapes and styles have changed
throughout history. And boy, have they changed. Influenced by everything from climate
conditions and superstitions to cultural values and religious beliefs, eyebrows reflect
more than the evolution of style—they reflect the evolution of humanity.

THE
ANCIENT BROW AGE
started with...

the egyptians

The ancient Egyptians created the earliest and most enduring style of makeup and eye adornment. When archaeologists and adventurers (think Indiana Jones) discovered the ancient tombs of the Egyptian pharaohs near the end of the nineteenth century, they unearthed a fashion surprise: The Egyptians loved their makeup.

AND IT WASN'T JUST THE WOMEN.

Ancient hieroglyphics on the walls of tombs clearly show both men and women wearing cosmetics to darken and accentuate the natural lines of the eye and brow. There were two colors of eye makeup at the time—green and black. The Egyptians used malachite, a green mineral that is a carbonate of copper, ground into a fine powder to add sparkle and color to the lower lid. Kohl (a black velvety powder made primarily from galena, a lead ore mineral) was used to accentuate and extend the line around the eyes and also to darken and enhance the brows, which might have been completely tweezed or shaved off.

BEAUTY POWER, PLEASE!

WEARING MALACHITE POWDER AROUND THE EYES WAS BELIEVED TO SUMMON THE POWER AND PROTECTION OF HATHOR, THE ANCIENT GODDESS OF BEAUTY, JOY, LOVE, AND WOMEN.

One of the best surviving examples of Egyptian brow beauty and face decoration from that era is the bust of Queen Nefertiti, Great Royal Wife of the pharaoh Akhenaten, who ruled Egypt around 1300 BCE. Her name translates as THE BEAUTY HAS COME. The bust reflects not only her perfectly symmetrical and proportional features but also ancient Egyptian makeup style at its best. Her brows were darkened dramatically, and her eyes were lined with kohl, extending the outer eye line to a point near the temple.

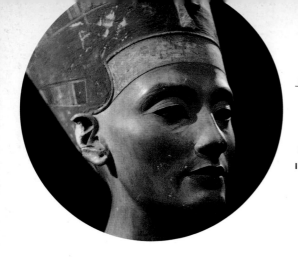

DURING AKHENATEN'S REIGN, NEFERTITI ENJOYED UNPRECEDENTED POWER. SOME SCHOLARS BELIEVE THAT SHE ACTUALLY RULED EGYPT FOR A BRIEF PERIOD FOLLOWING THE DEATH OF HER HUSBAND.

THE ANCIENT EGYPTIANS PRIZED THEIR BROW AND EYE COSMETICS then as much as makeup lovers do today. How do we know? They took their brow beautifiers to the grave—and it wasn't just the pharaohs or the very wealthy who did. Archaeologists have found remains of simple cosmetic pots and other eye-color containers, such as leather pouches, conch shells, and hollow reeds, in even the most modest ancient graves.

Cosmetics jars and boxes owned by Egyptian rulers or the wealthy classes were ornate and elaborately decorated, often carved into the shapes of beloved animals, such as bears and swans.

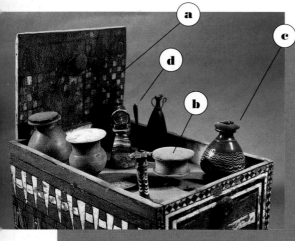

The contents of this ancient Egyptian cosmetics box look surprisingly similar to the jars, pots, and bottles of lotions and potions on a modern woman's vanity.

QUITE THE VANITY CASE

In ancient Egypt, beauty rituals began at an early age and continued into the afterlife, judging from the fully loaded cosmetics boxes buried beside their owners. Hey, you never know who you might meet on the other side!

a. The ornately decorated box was typically made of ivory, ebony, or wood.

b. Tiny clay pot for healing ointment or salve.

c. Petite ceramic urns contained kohl or malachite powder.

d. Handmade tool for applying kohl to brows and around the eyes.

the power of KOHL

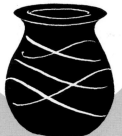

The kohl eye makeup worn by the ancient Egyptians was not just ornamental or reflective of a desire for greater beauty; it also served practical and medicinal purposes and even played a role in spiritual practices. The strongest evidence for this is that *everyone* in ancient Egypt wore kohl around the eyes, regardless of gender, age, or class.

Experts theorize that Egyptians believed that wearing kohl around the eye area was very powerful. Kohl could:

- *Shield the eyes from the harsh sun by absorbing light rays (just like that war paint pro football players wear today)*

- *Cure various eye diseases*

- *Keep flies away to guard against future disease*

- *Protect from being cursed by the Evil Eye*

In ancient Egypt, an unadorned eye was considered unprotected—and vulnerable to the Evil Eye. (This was seriously bad news, causing a lifetime of horrible luck and, quite possibly, hysterical blindness.) Mothers would apply kohl to their children's and even their infant's eyes to strengthen the eyes and protect their kids from being cursed. In rural parts of Egypt, mothers still do this.

KOHL FUEL—NOT JUST DECORATIVE!

IN 2010 FRENCH SCIENTISTS REPORTED RESEARCH INDICATING THAT THE KOHL MAKEUP WORN BY THE ANCIENT EGYPTIANS DID HAVE REAL MEDICINAL BENEFITS. GALENA, THE LEAD ORE MINERAL USED IN KOHL, CAN BOOST THE IMMUNE SYSTEM AND GUARD AGAINST INFECTION BY STIMULATING THE PRODUCTION OF NITRIC OXIDE.

ONE RECIPE

for

Ancient

Egyptian

KOHL

- Pound galena crystals with gum and frankincense; then mix with goose fat.

- Fold in cow dung, and burn to release the lead oxide.

- Mix with milk and fresh rainwater until you have a smooth, sooty goop.

- Pound again in a mortar.

- Decant several times to remove excess liquid.

- When the kohl is reduced to a fine velvety powder, it's ready!

Apply around the eyes and over your brows with a smooth, rounded stick or a flattened piece of wood, metal, or bone. Be sure to store your kohl in a decorative bowl or pot—and take it with you wherever you go!

it wasn't just
the Egyptians!

Here are some other Brow Age discoveries—
evidence that everyone in the ancient Mediterranean was doing it!

- *Following the reign of the Medes in Persia, kings carried their personal cosmetics cases—containing kohl and tweezers—with them into battle.*

- *Ancient Cretan frescoes (circa 500 BCE) show women with thin black eyebrows drawn into elegant, idealized shapes.*

- *To enhance and blacken the brow, the Sumerians were known to use a blend of galena and lampblack (soot from an oil lamp or other flame) mixed with vegetable resin and animal fat.*

- *The Assyrians used antimony (a soft metal ground into a lustrous silvery white powder) to decorate their eyelashes and brows.*

- *A cosmetics pot made of malachite and gold was discovered in a Sumerian tomb. Its contents? A tiny spoon (most likely for scooping and applying cosmetic powder or paste) and a mini pair of tweezers.*

- *Evidence of kohl used as an eye and brow cosmetic has turned up in the Middle East, North Africa, the Horn of Africa, and Southeast Asia. There is a word for kohl in more than fifteen different languages. In Arabic, the literal meaning of the word kohl is to brighten the eyes.*

The Brow Age continues . . .

THE *Ancient Mediterranean:*
A HOT SPOT
IN BROW HISTORY

the greeks

In ancient Greece, no self-respecting woman from a good family would be caught dead wearing makeup. Although women were treated more like the property of men than like individuals with rights, there was still an expectation of female purity, even among married women. Courtesans, the working girls of the day, were the only women to decorate the face and eyes. They darkened their brows and lined their eyelids with a delicate but distinct line drawn with a brush dipped in black incense. Yep, the world's first liquid eyeliner!

Unlike today—and just about every other era—the unibrow on a woman was seen as a symbol of great intelligence and beauty. The unibrow was so prized that women would often fill in the gap between their brows with kohl or black paint. And if that wasn't enough, truly enterprising and intelligent beauties wore *false* eyebrows made of dyed goat hair, introducing another first: the eyebrow wig.

the romans

Unlike the typical Greek woman, the Roman woman had it going on. Women of means were slaves to fashion—but nothing else. They had style, power, and freedom, often living separately from their husbands. It was a time of luxury and decadence, especially among the wealthy and the ruling class. The style of the day for women translated into elaborate fashion, jewelry, and cosmetic adornments. Roman women lightened their faces, wore perfume and wigs, dyed their hair blond, and painted their faces and eyes. A woman without makeup was considered quite plain and poor. And it wasn't just the women who loved their cosmetics—the men loved them, too.

Just like the Greeks, the Romans found great beauty and value in a woman's unibrow. They, too, filled in the natural space between the brows and used brow wigs to create the effect of unibrow beauty. It would not have been uncommon for a wealthy Roman woman to have an entire cosmetics box filled with false eyebrows—which, of course, she would never let anyone see. (Some things really haven't changed.)

the middle brow ages

In medieval times, the brow took a turn for the worse.

It was a new world with a new economy—basically, no economy. Just about everyone was a peasant, and personal hygiene plunged to an all-time low. In the early Middle Ages, no one had time to think about their eyebrows. Regardless of class, everyone was too busy fighting for their lives—dodging Barbarian invasions and attacks from starving neighboring villagers, plagues, famines, and other fun stuff—at least in Europe. These were tough times for everyone, and it showed in the untouched brows.

NEWS OF THE EYEBROW BEGAN TO EMERGE AROUND THE EARLY 1300s.

The new ideal of beauty for women was virginal innocence, influenced by the Catholic Church, the dominant and unifying cultural force in Europe at that time. Extremely pale skin became a symbol of a woman's purity as well as a sign of wealth and nobility. It was all the rage.

To achieve this look, upper-class women began painting their faces ghost-white with a variety of concoctions. The most common was ceruse, a blend of white lead and vinegar. A layer of this white paint smoothed over the face, neck, and bosom not only created the ideal whiteness, but it also concealed skin problems and pox, which was common at the time. Some women went so far as to add pale blue fake veins over their whitened skin, along with a bit of rouge to their lips and a trace of kohl around the eyes.

For women of means, the beauty regimen might also have included frequent visits to the barber/surgeon, who would pluck, trim, or shave all unwanted facial hair and then open a vein to bleed out just enough blood to create that naturally-pale-but-not-yet-dead look. **(AND YOU THINK GOING TO THE SPA/SALON ON A REGULAR BASIS NOW IS TOUGH!)**

high brow fashion

Medieval women also had begun shaving off their brows completely or tweezing them into a very thin, very high, closer-to-God arch. But it wasn't just the eyebrows that had to go. Women removed any facial hair (and other body hair) that might suggest sexual maturity rather than purity, and they even shaved or tweezed the hairline to convey childlike innocence, devoid of any sexuality, and to emulate the high hairlines of aristocracy and royalty.

Portraits of Queen Elizabeth I, who ruled England and Ireland from 1558 until her death in 1603, offer excellent examples of the prevailing standard of beauty in the late Middle Ages. Her brows appear so faint in some paintings that they may actually have been completely shaved off.

DEATH BECOMES HER

THE SLATHERING OF TOXIC LEAD-BASED PAINT ALL OVER THE SKIN PROVED TO NOT HAVE A GOOD LONG-TERM EFFECT ON ONE'S LOOKS. ACCORDING TO ONE AUTHOR, OVER TIME THE SKIN BEGAN TO APPEAR GRAY AND SHRIVELED. A NUMBER OF HISTORIANS HAVE THEORIZED THAT THE DEATH OF QUEEN ELIZABETH I MAY HAVE BEEN CAUSED BY LEAD POISONING FROM HER DAILY USE OF CERUSE MAKEUP.

OH, WHAT PRICE BEAUTY!

COSMETICS AND THE SIN OF ADULTERY

IN THE THIRTEENTH CENTURY, WHEN THOMAS AQUINAS, THE GREAT ITALIAN PRIEST, THEOLOGIAN, AND PHILOSOPHER, WAS ASKED ABOUT THE ETHICS OF WOMEN WEARING COSMETICS, HIS ANSWER WAS BOTH CLEAR AND WIDE OPEN TO INTERPRETATION. A WOMAN SHOULD MAKE HERSELF ATTRACTIVE ENOUGH THAT HER HUSBAND WOULD NOT STRAY AND COMMIT THE SIN OF ADULTERY, BUT NOT SO ATTRACTIVE THAT SHE MIGHT DRAW THE EYE OF OTHER WOMEN'S HUSBANDS.

WAIT. IS THAT TWO FINGERFULS OF CERUSE OR THREE?

This desire for a look of virginal purity, combined with generally poor nutrition and a lot of time in those dark, dank castles and walled cities, left medieval women looking rather unhealthy. In fact, the prevailing look for aristocratic women was decidedly egglike. But apparently the **NOBLEMEN AND KNIGHTS WERE INTO IT.** (And the clergy definitely approved.)

The invention of the mirror began to change all that. When women discovered they could see themselves in pieces of highly polished silver, the mirrors of the day, they realized there was grooming to be done. We can see abundant evidence of this return to an appreciation of beauty in Renaissance art.

MEANWHILE, IN OTHER NEWS . . .

IN OTHER CULTURES BEYOND EUROPE, DECORATING THE EYES AND FACE DURING THE MIDDLE AGES WAS STILL A GO. ARTWORK AND MOSAICS FROM THIS PERIOD SHOW THAT THE BOLD, BEAUTIFUL UNIBROW ON WOMEN WAS STILL LOVED, AND EYES RIMMED WITH KOHL CONTINUED TO FLOURISH IN THE BYZANTINE EMPIRE IN THE NORTHERN MEDITERRANEAN AS WELL AS IN ITALY.

news to amuse from around the brow world

RUSSIA For superstitious Russians, long eyebrows are loaded with hidden meaning—they mean you're a wizard!

CHINA Long eyebrows are universally considered a sign of good fortune.

MEXICO Fashionable brow trends are set by an unlikely source—highly dramatic eyebrows on the actresses in *telenovelas*, those wildly popular soap opera–like mini-series. Can you say, **"IS THAT A MACHETE IN YOUR POCKET, OR ARE YOU JUST HAPPY TO SEE ME? I WANT TO KISS YOU MADLY, BUT YOU MIGHT BE THE EVIL IDENTICAL TWIN OF MY LONG-LOST LOVE FROM THE DEEPLY TROUBLED YOUTH WING OF THE CONVENT"** in Spanish with just your eyebrows? Come on, sure you can!

BROW HIGHLIGHTS

of the Sixteenth, Seventeenth, Eighteenth, and Nineteenth Centuries

MID-16TH CENTURY

In England, masks become a favorite party favor for men and women among the gentry. Great for flirting and easy on the eyebrows. Brows were unseen and left untouched.

WAY, WAY BACK

Sometime way back when, the unibrow on babes fell out of fashion, and threading, an ancient art of removing brow hair with cotton thread, was born. The exact birthplace is unclear. Threading may have originated in Turkey, India, Persia, or East Asia. Today it thrives in India.

LATE 16TH CENTURY

Renaissance painters in the Golden Age of Venice captured the beauty of Italian women—long, flowing bleached-blond hair and perfectly arched brows.

WAY BACK

The earliest form of waxing goes all the way back to ancient Egyptian times, when women used a sticky mix of oil and honey to remove unwanted hair. Later, the Greeks used resin or tree pitch. Thank goodness for progress—and modern moisturizing wax!

CIRCA 1700

In France, women of the court painted their faces white (even adding faux blue veins). Brows had to be penciled in over the white paint.

EARLY/MID-18TH CENTURY

Personal care and hygiene were on the rise! We find the first evidence of breath fresheners and the first known depilatory for facial hair (a hair-raising paste made of smashed eggshells mixed with water).

MID-18TH CENTURY

Copying the styles of Kabuki theater, Japanese courtesans shaved their brows, applied white paint to their faces, and reapplied the brows with a delicate brush.

In Western Europe, full eyebrows were an absolute must for upper-class beauties and courtiers. If the brows didn't come naturally, not a problem—a lovely piece of mouse hide adhered to the forehead would do, and often did!

EARLY 18TH CENTURY

For a change, the only women in England *not* decorating their faces and tweezing their brows were the prostitutes.

LATE 18TH CENTURY

Commercial cosmetics were not yet on the scene. Women used burned matchsticks to darken their brows and lashes.

EARLY 19TH CENTURY

Among the fashionable English, the use of cosmetics was considered a tacky attempt at deception. Eyes were free of any adornment, and brows were allowed to grow wild.

Crazy EYEBROW INVENTIONS!

The eyebrow—and methods for improving its health and happiness—has captured the imagination of great thinkers for decades. Based on these patented product ideas, genius and insanity are often just a hair's width apart.

a **EYEBROW COVER ELEMENT** Tired of looking at your boring old hairy eyebrows? Dying to cover them completely and add ornaments, gemstones, or precious metals that coordinate with your rings, bracelets, and brooches? You're in luck! The Eyebrow Cover Element patent has been approved.

PATENT NUMBER: **4,942,891**
PATENT DATE: **JULY 24, 1990**
INVENTOR'S HOME COUNTRY: **ITALY**

b **EYEBROW SHAVING APPARATUS** Want to shave your eyebrows with what looks like a small bent Popsicle stick with one, or preferably two, exposed blades and is described as "relatively safe in use"? Uh, no thanks.

PATENT NUMBER: **4,961,262**
PATENT DATE: **OCTOBER 9, 1990**
INVENTOR'S HOME STATE: **CALIFORNIA**

c **EYEBROW CURLER** Are flat, limp eyebrows keeping you down? Do you dream of brows that curl up toward the sky, just like your lashes? Then this one's for you! When the serrated upper jaw meets the smooth lower jaw in a big chomp-down on your brows, you'll be in curly-brow heaven.

PATENT NUMBER: **3,339,561**
PATENT DATE: **SEPTEMBER 5, 1967**
INVENTOR'S HOME STATE: **CALIFORNIA**

d **EYEBROW SHIELD** Is tossing and turning at night wearing away your eyebrows? Do you wake up in the morning and find more brows on your pillow than on your face? At last, there's hope. The amazing Eyebrow Shield offers two concave protective covers made of stiff leather, metal, rubber, or celluloid, held in place by an elastic headband around the back of the head. A central band goes over the top of the head to stabilize the Eye Shield while you slumber in comfort. Oh yeah, there's also a fetching under-the-chin strap that ties around the back of the neck. So far, nighttime strangulation has not been a problem. Added bonus: It's a fail-safe birth control device.

PATENT NUMBER: **1,055,382**
PATENT DATE: **MARCH 11, 1913**
INVENTOR'S HOME STATE: **ILLINOIS**

ARCH
of the brow in the twentieth century

IN THE BEGINNING OF THE CENTURY, naturalism emerged as the dominant fashion. Most women tossed their corsets aside and let their hair and brows grow wild as they frolicked, Bohemian style, through the woods. Only the very wealthy—heiresses, duchesses, and queens—tended their brows or even wore eye makeup, and then only at night.

THE 1910s ushered in an exciting new influence: theatrical makeup. When the Ballets Russes arrived in Paris for the first time, the troupe members' dark and dramatic eyeliner mesmerized fashion and beauty leaders in Europe. The Russians ignited the first sparks of a big trend: the return to dark, kohl-lined eyes. When silent-film star Theda Bara played the title role in *Cleopatra* (1917), the heavy use of kohl around the eyes took off in the United States and continued into the 1920s.

THE 1920s was a time of fashion, freedom, and fun. Flappers and films stars such as Clara Bow—known as the "It Girl"—and Louise Brooks cut their hair boldly short, and just about everyone followed. Shorter bangs focused more attention on the brows. And that new thing called the film industry focused the world on Hollywood fashion and style. Its influence, guided by Max Factor and other top makeup artists, was fast and furious. The extremely thin, arched brow became the new symbol of sex appeal and sophistication.

THE 1930s followed the crash of the stock market. During the Great Depression, money was tight, and so were eyebrows. Most women kept their brows neat and trim, with soft arches. Perhaps eyebrows were the only thing women felt they could control in those uncertain times, or perhaps tweezing was the only entertainment most could afford. Film stars such as Marlene Dietrich, Claudette Colbert, and Jean Harlowe tweezed their brows into thin, high, glamorous arches. When Vivian Leigh played Scarlet O'Hara in the 1939 film *Gone with the Wind*, she bucked the brow trend. Unlike other women in the film, Leigh refused to tweeze her brows skinny because she thought they were essential to her ability to express emotion on camera.

The Mexican painter Frida Kahlo featured—and even exaggerated—her dark unibrow in many of her self-portraits. She didn't exactly start a unibrow trend, but she did earn respect as a serious female painter with a serious love of female facial hair.

THE 1940s and World War II changed women's roles and identities in a flash. Not only did women have to run their households alone while their husbands were off fighting, but many were also called into the workplace to fill the industrial jobs formerly held by men. It was a time that ignited independence and personal strength in many American women. Rosie the Riveter, a character introduced by the US government to inspire women to join the workforce, says it all: I've got a strong body *and* strong brows. Basically, she was too busy working to spend much time shaping her eyebrows.

The end of the war saw a quick return to fashion and femininity. Sales at cosmetics counters surged, and corsets were worn tighter to accentuate the female form. During this time, *Vogue* began to offer beauty advice to readers and prominently featured the well-shaped brow on its covers.

THE 1950s reflected a return to all things feminine. A renewed focus on grace and beauty meant that eyebrows got a lot of attention and were usually shaped into delicate arches, then accentuated with dark powder. The ideal brow was full and soft and shapely—like the rest of a woman's body. For the first time, the eyebrow was considered more than just an eye accessory or a frame for the face. It was—all on its own—a thing of beauty.

THE 1960s echoed the freedom, rebellion, and creativity of the 1920s. But it was a decade split in two. For some people, the 1950s never ended. The prevailing style remained neat, polished, ladylike, and conservative (think Jackie Kennedy). For others, generally of the younger generation, the '60s was one big psychedelic party (think Twiggy). Rock and roll took off, bold patterns and prints dominated fashion, hippies were protesting, and most people wanted to make love, not war. The eyebrow got a little lost in all the craziness, taking a backseat to wild hair, eyes with thick, black eyeliner (liquid eyeliner had just been invented), and long eyelashes, especially long false lashes. Brows were minimized—or completely ignored—so that they wouldn't clash with the eyes.

WHEN ELIZABETH TAYLOR PLAYED CLEOPATRA IN THE 1963 FILM, TREND EXPERTS PREDICTED A WIDE RESURGENCE IN HEAVY KOHL EYELINER AND THICK, DARK EYEBROWS. WRONG. THE BEHIND-THE-SCENES DRAMA BETWEEN ELIZA-BETH TAYLOR AND RICHARD BURTON (THEY FELL IN LOVE AND LEFT THEIR SPOUSES) WAS FAR MORE DRAMATIC AND INTERESTING TO THE PUBLIC THAN THE DRAMA ONSCREEN. THE RESULT WAS THE OPPOSITE OF WHAT HAD BEEN PREDICTED. WHEN MOST WOMEN LEFT THE THEATERS, THEY WEREN'T THINK-ING ABOUT BOLD, BEAUTIFUL CLEOPATRA; THEY WERE THINKING *LIZ TAYLOR REALLY NEEDS TO RUN HOME AND GROOM HER BROWS—AND SO DO I!*

THE 1970s were fun—but not the best time for eyebrows. The women's rights movement was gaining momentum, and unfortunately, so was disco. Things that sparkled, shimmied, and shined were all the rage. Glitter. Polyester. Lamé. It wasn't pretty. Eyebrows were either tweezed into unnatural shapes and sizes and dusted with reflective powders, or completely ignored under a wild mane of feathered hair. But not in San Francisco, where a whole new brow happening was happening.✳

✳ THE ADDED BENEFIT

In 1976 Jean and Jane Ford, fashion-setting twin sisters from Indiana, opened a hip little shop called the Face Place in the Mission District of San Francisco. This makeup, brow-shaping, and beauty boutique became a destination hot spot for women who wanted to look great and have a blast doing it. That fun, face-loving concept, combined with beauty formulas that really worked and packaging that made women laugh, was the spark that ignited Benefit Cosmetics.

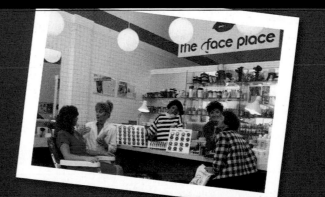

THE 1980s was a decade of prosperity and abundance. Greed was good. Everyone wanted more. Unfortunately for women, that translated into big hair, big shoulder pads, and big, bushy eyebrows. The hottest actors, models, and performers of the decade—Brooke Shields, Cindy Crawford, Isabella Rossellini, Kelly McGillis, Madonna—all had big, thick, free-range brows. The look was big, bold, beautiful—and completely natural. It took off and set the trend among models, actors, and the public for the entire decade.

THE 1990s saw the growth of personal expression through makeup. More and more branded cosmetics counters were popping up in department stores—and not just in the big cities. Women everywhere became their own personal makeup artists. In general, brows got more loving care and were better groomed. But styles were all over the brow map and open to interpretation. One fashion designer pushed thick manly brows, while another promoted a '70s-retro thin, rounded arch. Madonna alone proved that—as long as it works with the rest of your look—anything goes in browtown.

THE **NOW BROW** IN THE

twenty-first century

Since the turn of the millennium, eyebrows have continued to thrive. Around the world, brows are recognized as an important part of any modern woman's beauty package. In growing numbers, even men are appreciating the importance of brows and heading fearlessly down the brow-grooming path.

Brow styles have held strong, staying naturally groomed and shapely. While styles do fluctuate a bit, often reflecting subtle cultural differences in countries or regions of the globe, one universal trend is clear: Eyebrows are **OBJECTS OF BEAUTY** and not to be ignored. Any woman who cares about her appearance—from the corporate executive to the soccer mom, prom queen, and got-it-going-on granny—keeps her brows in shape and looking fabulous. And now, with brow salons and spas popping up all over, it's never been easier to get your brows groomed by a pro. Frankly, getting your brows done is the new manicure. It used to be a treat or a splurge for special occasions.

Now it's a modern beauty must!

NOW THAT EYEBROWS HAVE HIT THE BIG TIME, IT MIGHT BE TIME TO TAKE BROW APPRECIATION TO THE NEXT LEVEL.

THE **browy** AWARDS

THE IMPORTANCE OF THE EYEBROW IN THE ARTS has been woefully underappreciated. But it's not too late to rectify that. For an outstanding eyebrow performance in a film, television, art, or life,

THE BROWY GOES TO . . .

THE LEADING WOMEN

MOST ALLURING PINK BROWS: MISS PIGGY

BEST BROWS TO SHARE THE STAGE WITH A DIVA HEADBAND:
WONDER WOMAN

SEXIEST UNGROOMED DUDE BROWS ON A GIRL:
BROOKE SHIELDS (CIRCA 1980)

BEST PERFORMANCE WITH NO EYEBROWS: IT'S A TIE!
DORA THE EXPLORER **AND** WHOOPI GOLDBERG

BEST FIFTEEN MINUTES OF EYEBROW FAME:
EDIE SEDGWICK, ANDY WARHOL'S MUSE AND SUPERSTAR

MOST DETERMINED-TO-SAVE-THE-WORLD BROWS ON A BLOND:
SARAH MICHELLE GELLAR AS BUFFY THE VAMPIRE SLAYER

BEST MUSEUM-QUALITY UNIBROW: FRIDA KAHLO

BEST COSMETICALLY ENHANCED BROW-JOB: PAMELA ANDERSON

BEST "I'M SO TOTALLY INNOCENT" BROW:
PARIS HILTON IN (ALL) HER MUG SHOTS

BEST MEOW! BROW CAT WOMAN:
ANN-MARGRET

THE LEADING MEN

BEST BROODING BROWS: MARLON BRANDO

LEAST TERRIFYING UNIBROW: BERT (*SESAME STREET*)

BEST CRAZY BROWS: JACK NICHOLSON (*THE SHINING*)

BEST DRAG QUEEN BROWS: DIVINE

MOST DISTINCTIVE BROWS
(WHICH PLAYED SECOND FIDDLE TO THE DISTINCTIVE EARS):
LEONARD NIMOY AS MR. SPOCK IN *STAR TREK*

BEST NESTABLE BROWS: BORIS KARLOFF

BEST ACHING-HEARTTHROB BROWS:
MONTGOMERY CLIFT

BEST MUSTACHE-LIKE BROW (LIVE ACTION): CLARK GABLE

SEXIEST DAD BROWS:
PETER GALLAGHER AS SANDY COHEN ON *THE O.C.*

BEST SANTA CLAUS BROWS THAT DOUBLE AS A COAT RACK:
ANDY ROONEY

BEST SITCOM-DISASTER BROWS:
SEINFELD'S UNCLE LEO WITH HIS DRAWN-ON PERMA-ANGRY BROWS

LET'S ALL RAISE A BROW to honor the rich and distinguished history of the eyebrow—and nod with solemn reverence at all it has accomplished through the ages. Now raise two brows and see what the future of the eyebrow holds for you!

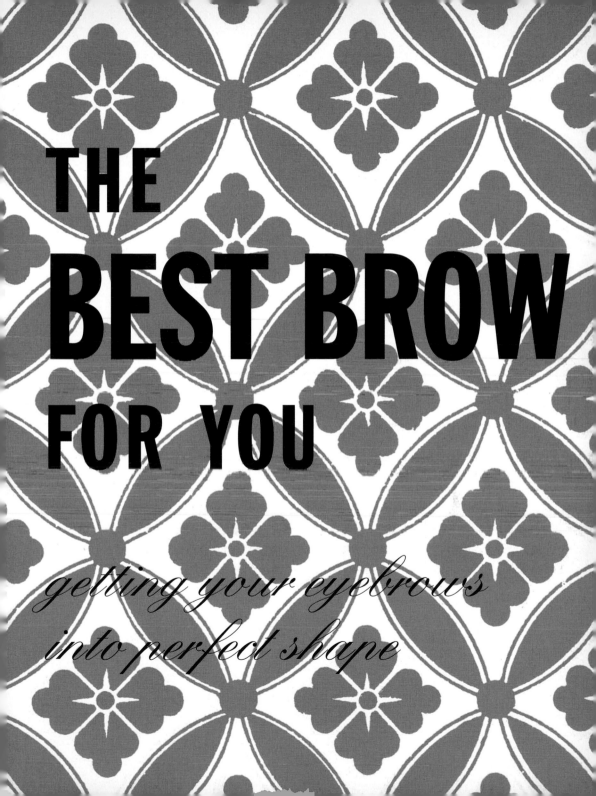

THE
BEST BROW
FOR YOU

getting your eyebrows into perfect shape

WE COVERED THE BASIC PRINCIPLES OF A WELL-GROOMED BROW in chapter 1, and in chapter 2 we learned some fascinating history. Now it's all about you. Here we get personal and focus on the specific elements you should evaluate when determining your best brow shape. (If you need a quick refresher on the basics, turn to page 25.)

When deciding on the best brow shape for you, there are two main things to think about: your eyebrow itself and your eyebrow within the context of your face.

Let's start with your eyebrow. The brow has four main characteristics:

● *shape*　　　● *thickness*　　　● *color*　　　● *length*

Any one of these four is open to change and improvement. The goal is to optimize all four so that they work together to create the best brow for your face.

First, let's get the terminology down.

THE **ANATOMY** OF A **BROW**

a　Start (your natural Point A)

b　Arch (your natural Point B)

c　End (your natural Point C)

d　Thickness

e　Height

f　Length

To locate your natural Points A, B, and C, see pages 25–26. To determine your best thickness, height, and length, look at what Mother Nature gave you!

Use the thickest part of your natural brow as a guide for how thick your brow should be from your natural Point A to Point B.

And how high or long should your brow be? Once you discover your natural Points A, B, and C, all will be revealed!

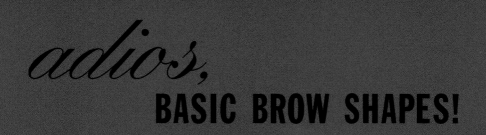

adios, BASIC BROW SHAPES!

In other books, you can read about "basic brow shapes." These shapes may have made sense to someone back in the day, but today? No. Unless you're making your eyebrows out of black electrical tape or entering a Lady Groucho Marx competition, they're not much help.

- *sharp angled*
- *soft angled*
- *rounded*
- *curved*
- *flat*

So ignore any basic shapes—**YOU'RE NOBODY'S BASIC.** Instead, all you need to look at is unique and beautiful *you.*

let's look at your whole face

If you've been staring at your brows in a huge magnifying mirror, now is a good time to get out from under the microscope and look at your brows in a regular mirror. You need to be able to see your eyebrows in the context of the rest of your face.

Before you can design the best brow shape for you, you should consider:

- *your face shape*
- *your eye shape*
- *your other features*
- *your personal style*

what shape is your face?

The shape of most faces falls into one of four categories:

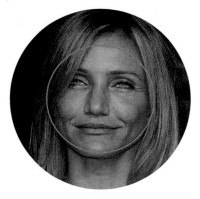

ROUND: Widest at the cheeks and nearly as wide as it is long.

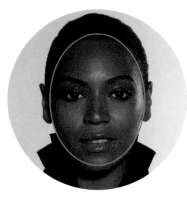

OVAL: Forehead, cheekbones, and jawline are all about the same width; jawline tapers to the chin.

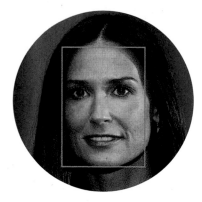

SQUARE: Forehead, cheekbones, and jawline are all about the same width; jawline is square and cuts a sharper angle to the chin.

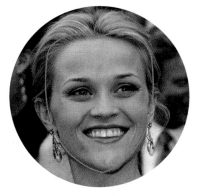

HEART: Forehead and cheekbones are about the same width and wider than the chin; cheekbones gently taper to the chin.

A WELL-SHAPED BROW can trick the eye into seeing less where there is more and more where there is less. (Oh, if only we had eyebrows on our butts . . .) Here are a few brow-shaping tips for creating the most flattering optical illusion for your face shape.

If your face shape is **ROUND** . . .

DO: enhance the natural angles in your brow and maximize the peak of your arch.

DON'T: shape your brow into a rounded arch. (It will just echo the shape of your face and make it appear rounder.)

If your face shape is **OVAL** . . .

DO: go for a strong, defined brow to complement the shape of your face.

DON'T: try a flat, thin brow. (It will make your face appear longer.)

If your face shape is **SQUARE** . . .

DO: try an angular brow with a well-defined arch. (The arch will draw attention up and away from your jaw.)

DON'T: go with a soft, rounded shape. (It won't have the strength to balance your face.)

If your face shape is **HEART** . . .

DO: shape your brow into a softer arch. (It will soften the point of your chin.)

DON'T: go with a straight, flat brow. (It will weigh your whole face down and make your forehead look even wider.)

JUST SAY NO to Stencils!

Using eyebrow stencils is the cookie-cutter approach to brow shaping. While some people still use them, they're old-school. A skilled brow expert will be able to shape your brows without ever using a stencil.

AND THINK ABOUT IT. Do you really want the shape of your brows to be modeled after a shape mass-produced in the eyebrow factory? Didn't think so. Just because it looked great on the face mannequin or on some movie star decades ago doesn't mean it will look good on your face now. The truth is, nature gave you everything you need to determine the best brow shape for you.

the feature story

Forget about your brows for a second and take a good look at your other features—your eyes, your nose, your lips, even your chin. What you're looking for is **BALANCE AND PROPORTION.** If you have small, refined features, you'll look best with thinner, more refined brows. If you have strong features or dark coloring, you'll need strong brows to balance the proportion of your strong features.

Here are a few rules of thumb to follow:

NATURE GAVE YOU	GOOD BROW PLAN	BAD BROW PLAN
LARGE EYES	strong and well-defined	thin and delicate
SMALL EYES	natural with a delicate arch	heavy or ungroomed
ALMOND-SHAPED EYES	angular with a high arch	overpowering or rounded
POINTED CHIN	natural with a subtle arch	flat or angular
HIGH CHEEKBONES	angled with a high arch	rounded or flat
HIGH FOREHEAD	full and angular with a high arch	flat or thin
NARROW FOREHEAD	flat with a slight arch	overpowering with a high arch

THE THIRD-EYE RULE

ACCORDING TO THE PREVAILING GODS AND GODDESSES OF BEAUTY PERFECTION (WHICH, OF COURSE, *ONLY* EXIST IN THEORY SOMEWHERE OFF IN BEAUTY NIRVANA), THE IDEAL DISTANCE BETWEEN THE EYES IS ABOUT ONE EYE WIDTH.

what's your SECRET BEAUTY WEAPON?

YEP. YOUR BROWS. If you have especially wide-set eyes, especially close-set eyes, or an especially broad nose, guess what: You also have an especially powerful secret beauty weapon to employ to offset those features—your eyebrows. By tweaking the start of your brows, you can trick the eye into seeing a more flattering view of you.

IF YOU HAVE CLOSE-SET EYES . . .

By moving the start of your brows (your natural Point A) out a teeny bit toward your temple to make more space between your brows, you can create the illusion of your eyes being set farther apart. Just like that—*open sesame!* (**NOTE TO BROW:** This is *not* something to experiment with at home. This is the time to get the help of a skilled professional.)

IF YOU HAVE WIDE-SET EYES . . .

If you cheat the start of your brow (your natural Point A) in toward the middle a tad, making your brows appear a bit closer together, you can create the illusion that your eyes are actually closer together, too. This is easy to achieve with a brow pencil or powder.

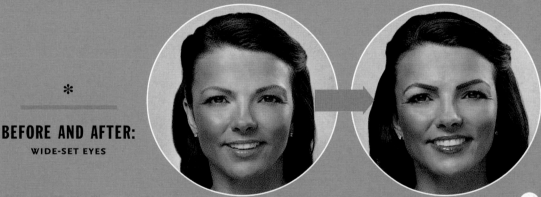

*

BEFORE AND AFTER:

WIDE-SET EYES

IF YOU HAVE A BROAD NOSE . . .

You may want to modify the basic principles we covered in chapter 1, on page 25. Instead of resting the pencil in the dimple where your nostril begins, try cheating it in toward the middle a bit to find the most flattering natural Point A for you.

*

BEFORE AND AFTER:
BROAD NOSE

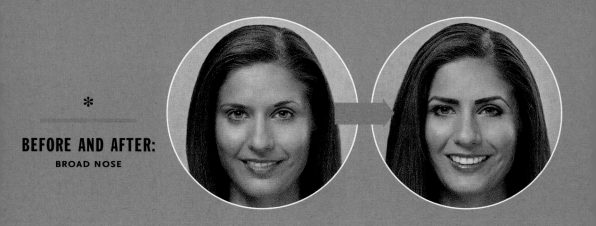

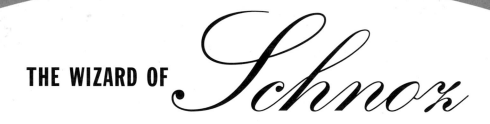

THE WIZARD OF *Schnoz*

If you have a prominent proboscis **(BIG NOSE)**, your eyebrows can work magic! They have special powers to create an optical illusion that minimizes your nose's appearance. Of course, there's nothing wrong with a prominent nose. In fact, some of the greatest beauties of all time are known for their standout noses. (Gisele, Barbra, Angelica, Sophia, Gaga, to name a few.) But if you don't do a little work to balance your features, a big nose can dominate your face, screaming, *look at me!* to everyone who sees. A strong nose on any face deserves strong, well-defined brows for balance—just like any diva on any stage deserves rockin' backup. When you get the balance just right, your brows will redirect other people's eyes, luring them away from your big, beautiful schnoz and right into your eyes.

your personality AND style

It's also smart to think about your personality and style (both in the sense of fashion and lifestyle) when determining the best brow for you. If you have a big personality, you can get away with bigger, bolder brows. If you're quiet and reserved, you probably don't want brows so bold that they overpower you. If your every move is graceful and elegant, your brows should be, too.

What do you do for a living? What do you typically wear to work? Are you conservative, liberal, undecided? Do you live in a big city? In the burbs? In the boonies?

THERE'S NO PERFECT RULE for how to factor your personality and personal style in to the brow-shaping equation. But you don't want your eyebrows to stand out or be in conflict with the rest of you. Think of it this way: The best brow for you makes you look great, works *with* your personal style, and lives happily in the world you've created for yourself.

Whatever your personality or style, when you walk into a room/gallery/barn, you want people to notice *you*—not your eyebrows. That's what a great brow shaping will do for you.

BREAKING THE BROW RULES

OF COURSE, THERE'S ALWAYS A TIME AND A PLACE FOR BREAKING THE RULES. BUT YOU HAVE TO KNOW THE RULES AND WHY THEY EXIST BEFORE YOU CAN BREAK THEM WISELY.

YOUR *best* BROW COLOR

Let's talk brow color for a minute. What's the best color for your eyebrows? It depends. A good general rule is to choose a brow color that matches the *deepest* shade of your hair color.

IF YOU HAVE LIGHT HAIR, go for the deepest shade you've got up top. (Blondes, that means your roots!)

IF YOU HAVE DARK HAIR, choose your deepest shade as well, *unless* your deepest shade is black. (Black brows can look very scary!) Opt for a dark brown instead—it's softer and more flattering.

If you're craving some HIGH BROW DRAMA, try one of these shades:

- *If your hair is platinum, stay close to your natural brow hair color while avoiding any warm tones.*
- *If your hair is silver, go for a cool, ash-blond shade.*
- *If you have truly black hair, go for a cool, deep taupe or brown— almost black but softer.*
- *If you're a redhead, follow the rules for light or dark hair, but choose a shade that's a touch more brown. (Orange brows are not allowed!)*

Of course, most rules are made to be broken, bent, tinted, and tweezed. Some blonds look great with dark brows, and some brunettes prefer a lighter, sun-kissed brow. Changing up the color of your brows is a great way to experiment with your look. Try a few different shades of pencil or powder on your brows. If you like what you see, you can take it outside. If you don't—no harm, no foul. Just wipe your brows clean and try something else, or stick with your natural color.

Even if you don't want to alter the color of your brows, you may still need to think about color before filling in sparse brows or adding definition with a pencil or powder. Choosing the right shade of product makes it easy to extend the end, heighten the arch, extend the inner corner, or make your brows appear thicker.

EYEBROW TINTING

IF YOU'VE CHANGED YOUR HAIR COLOR OR YOUR BROWS ARE FADING A BIT AS YOU GROW WISER— OR YOU JUST WANT TO TRY SOMETHING NEW—CHECK OUT EYEBROW TINTING AT YOUR FAVORITE BROW SPOT. IT'S A GREAT OPTION FOR CHANGING THE COLOR OF YOUR EYEBROWS WITH LASTING RESULTS. SAFE, GENTLE NATURAL DYES ARE USED TO ADJUST THE COLOR OF YOUR BROWS WHILE YOU SIT BACK AND RELAX OR RECLINE IN COMFORT. A BROW-TINTING TREATMENT COSTS ABOUT $25, AND THE COLOR STAYS STRONG FOR UP TO FOUR WEEKS.

BE SURE TO GET YOUR BROWS TINTED BY A PRO.

COLOR CORRECTION ALERT!

YOUR BEAUTY-OBSESSED FRIEND/SISTER/ROOMMATE JUST SAW SOMETHING ON TV/YOUTUBE/A WEBSITE ABOUT BROW BLEACHING AND TINTING. SHE'S CURIOUS—AND YOU'RE HER FIRST LUCKY CUSTOMER. STOP RIGHT THERE! IF YOU'RE CONSIDERING BLEACHING YOUR BROWS OR TINTING THEM WITH DYE, GET YOURSELF TO A HIGHLY TRAINED EXPERT! THIS IS NOT SOMETHING TO MESS WITH AT HOME.

SERIOUSLY. FOR REALS.

EYEBROW TRENDS

EVERY NOW AND THEN, A MODEL, FASHION DESIGNER, SINGER, OR ACTOR INTRODUCES SOME CRAZY NEW LOOK FOR EYEBROWS. ENJOY IT FOR WHAT IT IS—FASHION THEATER—AND APPRECIATE IT FROM A DISTANCE. UNLESS YOU'RE A PERFORMANCE ARTIST OR APPLYING TO CLOWN COLLEGE, YOU REALLY DON'T WANT TO FOLLOW ANY CRAZY BROW TRENDS. STICK TO WHAT WORKS FOR YOU AND LOOKS GREAT ON YOUR FACE.

THE ULTRATHIN BROW . . . WEARER BEWARE!

IT WAS ALL THE RAGE IN THE 1930s. BUT THE TRUTH IS, FEW WOMEN LOOK GOOD WITH A PENCIL-THIN, ARCHED BROW. IT'S SEVERE ON ANYONE, AND IT CAN EVEN MAKE YOU APPEAR HARD, MEAN, AND MUCH OLDER. AN ULTRATHIN BROW IS SO STYLIZED THAT YOU REALLY HAVE TO COMMIT YOUR WHOLE LOOK—CLOTHES, HAIR, AND MAKEUP—TO THAT STYLE TO PULL IT OFF, NOT TO MENTION THE TIME COMMITMENT. WITH ALL THE HOURS YOU'D HAVE TO SPEND IN FRONT OF A MIRROR TWEEZING TO KEEP THOSE THIN ARCHES IN SHAPE, YOU COULD WRITE A NOVEL OR GET AN ADVANCED DEGREE. IF YOU DO TRY IT, JUST KNOW WHAT YOU'RE GETTING INTO AND UNDERSTAND THAT IT'S A BIG COMMITMENT. AND BE SURE TO UNDERSTAND THAT OVERPLUCKING FOR A LONG PERIOD OF TIME CAN RESULT IN PERMANENT BROW-HAIR LOSS.

YOU'RE NEVER TOO OLD FOR

Great Brows!

As women age, their eyebrows tend to lose definition. It's frustrating. But it's natural and happens to just about everyone. The color of each hair lightens as the pigment within the inner shaft fades. The actual number of hairs in each brow also diminishes significantly over time. The result is washed-out brows, thinning brows, or maybe even no brows at all.

That's the bad news. Fortunately, **THERE'S GOOD NEWS, TOO.**

It's fast and easy to restore your brows to their best shape. All you need is tinted brow wax and powder to add color and definition, and you can finish with brow gel to add shine and texture that holds. Here's the best part: by cheating your natural brow line up a tad from the arch (Point B) to the end (Point C), you can achieve the effect of an instant, surgery-free eye-lift.

KEEP IN MIND THAT YOUR BEST BROWS IN YOUR FIFTIES AND SIXTIES ARE NOT THE SAME AS YOUR BEST BROWS IN YOUR TWENTIES AND THIRTIES. You still need to look at the proportion and balance of your face when designing your best brow shape. Pay special attention to your hair. Whether you're coloring your hair or going gray naturally, your hair color does change as you get older—and so should your brow color. The last thing you want to do is overaccentuate your eyebrows and end up looking like a caricature of yourself or worse—like Joan Crawford on a bender.

✳

BEFORE AND AFTER:
MATURE BROWS

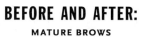

65

IN BROW YEARS, YOU LOOK . . .

FADED, WASHED-OUT EYEBROWS ARE AN INSTANT GIVEAWAY TO A WOMAN'S AGE. BY ADDING COLOR, DEFINITION, AND SHAPE TO YOUR BROWS, YOU CAN TAKE TEN YEARS OFF YOUR FACE IN MINUTES!

AND THEN THERE WERE NONE

IF YOU'VE NEVER HAD EYEBROWS, OR IF YOU'VE LOST THEM AS A RESULT OF OVERTWEEZING, ILLNESS, SURGERY, CHEMOTHERAPY, OR ANY OTHER TYPE OF TRAUMA, YOU DO HAVE OPTIONS FOR RE-CREATING NATURAL-LOOKING BROWS. LEARNING TO PENCIL IN YOUR BROWS ARTFULLY IS THE LEAST EXPENSIVE SOLUTION—BUT PENCIL DOES WASH OFF WHEN YOU SHOWER OR BATHE, SO YOU'LL STILL WAKE UP WITHOUT ANY EYEBROWS. YOU MAY WANT TO INVESTIGATE EYEBROW WIGS (THE BEST ONES LOOK SURPRISINGLY REAL!), EYEBROW TRANSPLANTS (EXPENSIVE BUT EFFEC-TIVE), OR EYEBROW TATTOOING. COSMETIC EYEBROW TATTOOING IS LIKE PERMANENT MAKEUP. INK THAT IS THE COLOR OF YOUR NATURAL HAIR IS INJECTED UNDER THE SKIN IN PATTERNS THAT SIMULATE REAL HAIR GROWTH. WHEN EYEBROW TATTOOING IS DONE BY A HIGHLY TRAINED EXPERT, THE RESULTS CAN LOOK AMAZING.

*

NOTE TO BROW:

ANYONE WHO INJECTS DYE OR INK UNDER THE SKIN IS PERFORM-ING THE FINE ART OF TATTOOING AND MUST BE LICENSED. BE SURE YOU ASK TO SEE PHOTOS OF THE PRACTITIONER'S WORK—AND THEIR LICENSE!—BEFORE ANYONE GETS NEAR YOU WITH A NEEDLE. IT'S NOT IMPOLITE TO ASK; IT'S JUST PLAIN SMART. P.S.: YOU ALSO MIGHT WANT TO CALL THREE FRIENDS AND TAKE A QUICK POLL BEFORE YOU GET YOUR BROWS TATTOOED. A TATTOO IS FOREVER, SO PROCEED WITH CAUTION.

GAME CHANGERS

A FEW EYEBROW OBSTACLES can change the basic rules for shaping your brows. Some are natural, some happen by accident, and some we ask for. All of them create a bit of a challenge. If you've got a mole, an eyebrow scar, or a brow piercing (or all three), here's how you can work with and around your unique body art to create the best brow shape for you.

MARVELOUS MOLES

If you have a mole in your eyebrow, it's a sign of **GOOD LUCK!** In the terminology of Mian Xiang, the ancient Chinese art of face reading, a hidden mole in the eyebrow is called *a pearl in the grass*. It's considered a sign of great talents waiting to be discovered. People who have this unique trait are usually intelligent and gifted individuals. According to Mian Xiang, if you have a *a pearl in the grass*, you also have successful siblings. You and your siblings like to work together to help one another become more successful. If your mole is pale or very big, then you may go through a difficult period when you are between thirty-one and thirty-four (oh, who doesn't?)—or suffer a serious injury during this time.

Unless your mole is quite large, **CHANCES ARE NO ONE BUT YOU EVEN NOTICES IT.** But if it catches your eye or bugs you in any way, there's an easy fix.

If the mole isn't darker than your skin color, go straight to the brow wax that best matches the color of your brow hairs. Add some brow color to the mole, and blend with the tip of your ring finger, patting gently so you don't rub the color off. Then finish with brow powder, applying with light, short strokes in the same direction as your hair growth. For symmetry, be sure to use brow wax and then powder on your other eyebrow as well. If the mole has pigment, you may want to start with a layer of concealer one shade deeper than your skin tone, then continue with the above makeup application technique.

Want more details right now on the best way to apply brow wax and powder for natural results? Turn to page 114.

MOLE ALERT!

IF YOUR MOLE HAS A HAIR GROWING OUT OF IT, **DO NOT** TWEEZE IT OUT! TWEEZING A HAIR FROM A MOLE CAN TRIGGER CELLULAR CHANGES WITHIN THE MOLE THAT MAY LEAD TO SKIN CANCER. THE BEST THING TO DO TO TAME THE WILD MOLE HAIR IS GET OUT YOUR NAIL SCISSORS AND TRIM IT— REGULARLY. IF YOUR MOLE IS ASYMMETRICAL, HAS IRREGULAR BORDERS, OR SEEMS TO BE CHANGING IN ANY WAY, HAVE IT CHECKED OUT IMMEDIATELY BY A DERMATOLOGIST.

SEXY SCARS

You were two, you were twelve, you were twenty-two. No one needs to know the details of how you got that sexy little slash of a scar that cuts through your eyebrow. If you love it as is, don't touch a thing. But if you want your scar to recede into your past and disappear into your fabulous new brows, then you can easily hide it. Just dab a little concealer (one shade deeper than the color of your scar) on the scar, press some brow powder on the scar, and then blend it in with the rest of your brow, brushing *with* the hair growth. You may also need to add some concealer above and below the scar to define a clean brow line.

PROUD PIERCINGS

OKAY, ADMIT IT. You got your brow pierced because you
wanted people to look at it. Success. Mission accomplished! Your
brow stands out, and so do you. Why is this a brow-shaping game changer? Well,
definitely for one reason and possibly for two.

ONE: Everybody *is* looking at your eyebrows—even more than usual, which is great!
So the pressure is on to keep your brows looking groomed and gorgeous. Grunge had
its moment, but let's be honest: A pierced, well-shaped brow on a woman is hot. A
pierced, furry brow is . . . yeah, going straight to hairy-dude belly button–ring land. If
you love your brow piercing (and you should!), wear it loud and proud—*and* be sure to
give your brows the care they deserve. It's a groom with a view!

TWO: Your pierced, well-groomed brow looks awesome, and so do you. Even so, there
may be a few occasions when you actually want to remove the hardware and kinda/
sorta/hopefully make the hole(s) thing completely disappear. You know, like when you
don't want to lose your future mother-in-law's complete adoration or that killer job
offer or your entire inheritance. (Shiny metal is the only thing Grandma can still see.
Why? *Why?!*) There's no shame in covering your shiny personal assets when necessary.

Here's how you do it:

● *Remove the hoop or stud.*

● *If the hole(s) is outside the actual eyebrow, try to fill it in with a pore mini-
mizer or blotting balm, then dab it with a concealer one shade deeper than
your skin color and blend, blend, blend. If the hole is in the actual brow, dab a
little tinted brow wax, then press some brow powder on it, and blend in with
the rest of your brow, brushing with the hair growth.*

EYEGLASSES HAVE SPECIAL POWERS. They are much more than corrective eye lenses with frames; they're face jewelry. They can be a cool accessory, a sexy prop—or both. You can flirt with them, through them, or over them. Glasses are fashion *and* function. But just because you wear glasses, that's no reason to ignore your eyebrows. Even the thickest glasses can't conceal your brows completely, and they sure don't replace your brows.

How could they? Glasses can't communicate your emotions or hint at what you're thinking.

They can't convey compassion or concern. They can't ponder or tease. They can't ask a probing question or doubt a tall tale. Glasses can't even look smart on their own. But you can look smart (and sexy!) wearing them—if you show your brows some love.

Think wearing glasses means there's no point in wearing eye makeup or grooming your brows? Think again! Glasses actually draw attention to your eye area, which makes it even *more* important to groom and define your brows. You don't have to do anything special—just follow the same brow mapping as anyone without glasses.

P.S.

THOSE GLASSES ARE COMING OFF AT SOME POINT!

know your options

By now you should have a really good idea of what needs to go so that you and your brows can look great. What's the best way to remove unwanted brow hairs? Well, it depends. Here are some things to consider:

1. How much brow hair do you want removed?

2. How much time do you have?

3. Do you have budget constrictions?

4. Do any other unique personal needs come to mind?

WAXING: This is by far the most effective, modern way to reshape your brows—for lots of reasons. It's fast, safe, relatively affordable, and fun—if you go to the right kind of brow bar. (Guess where! Yep. Benefit!) A highly trained professional maps out the best brow shape for you, then in small sections applies thin layers of warm wax and places strips of muslin cloth on top. The wax cools for a few seconds, essentially shrink-wrapping each hair for a superfirm grip. And—quick tug!—adios, unwanted brow hair.

TWEEZING: Great for removing stragglers and free-range brow hairs. If done correctly, tweezing can be as effective as waxing. It just takes a lot longer, since the hairs are removed one by one. If you have extremely sensitive skin or are taking any medication, tweezing can be a good choice. (See page 88 for more details on how medications affect the skin.)

TRIMMING: You can't reshape a brow by trimming alone. (Trimming should complement another form of hair removal such as waxing.) If you have thick, bushy brows or wild ones, trimming is for you—but it should never be done by you! See a professional. It's shockingly easy to cut your brows too short if you aren't an expert. And crew-cut brows . . . not a good look.

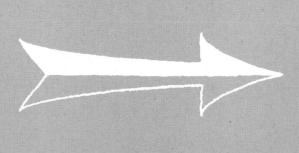

ELECTROLYSIS: Ouch! It's like electroshock therapy to the hair follicle. It works, but it hurts. After repeat treatments, electrolysis can effectively scramble the brain of each hair follicle so that it actually stops growing for good. A license is always required.

THREADING: It's an ancient art but not state of the art. Cotton threads are twisted and repeatedly pulled across the surface of the skin, catching, snapping, and removing hairs as they go. Some women love it, especially women with very dark, very thick brow hair, because you can do it weekly if needed. Unlike other methods of hair removal, threading is unregulated, so no one is licensed, which means health and hygiene are on the honor system.

SHAVING: Oh, please. There are much better ways! Shaving doesn't remove the entire hair like waxing or threading does. It just cuts the hair at the surface, leaving it right under the surface—often visible—and ready to grow out the next day. Leave all face shaving to the guys!

DEPILATORIES: Don't even think about it! Never, ever, *ever* use a depilatory (hair dissolving lotion or cream) to remove eyebrow hair—unless you actually want to go blind.

SUGARING: This is the primitive and much older (like a few thousand years older!) cousin of waxing. A lukewarm paste made of sugar, lemon juice, and water is applied over the unwanted hairs, then flicked off with a fingertip, removing the hairs—at least most of them. The process is similar to waxing but usually takes longer because it has to be done repeatedly to remove all the unwanted hair.

CONGRATULATIONS!

You've learned the brow basics, examined the shape of your eyebrows, and evaluated their health and happiness within the context of your face. If you're like most women, you've a discovered real opportunity for personal brow improvement. You understand the brow-shaping options *and* how to create the best brow shape for you. At last! You're ready to transform your now brows into wow brows.

STEP AWAY FROM THE MIRROR!

Whether you're looking for a major brow makeover or a little brow R&D (refine and define), this is the time for professional help. It's so worth it to take the time and spend the money to see a brow expert at a salon or brow spa*—at least once. A professional brow shaping is the safest, fastest, smartest way to get the best brow for you.

---

*

THE ADDED BENEFIT

And now, a word from our sponsor. Why go to just any brow salon when you can go to a Benefit Brow Bar or Boutique? Come on, they are the eyebrow experts. Benefit not only knows everything about brows and how to make them beautiful—they also make brows fun. Don't even try to deny it. It's page 73, and you're still holding this book!

4

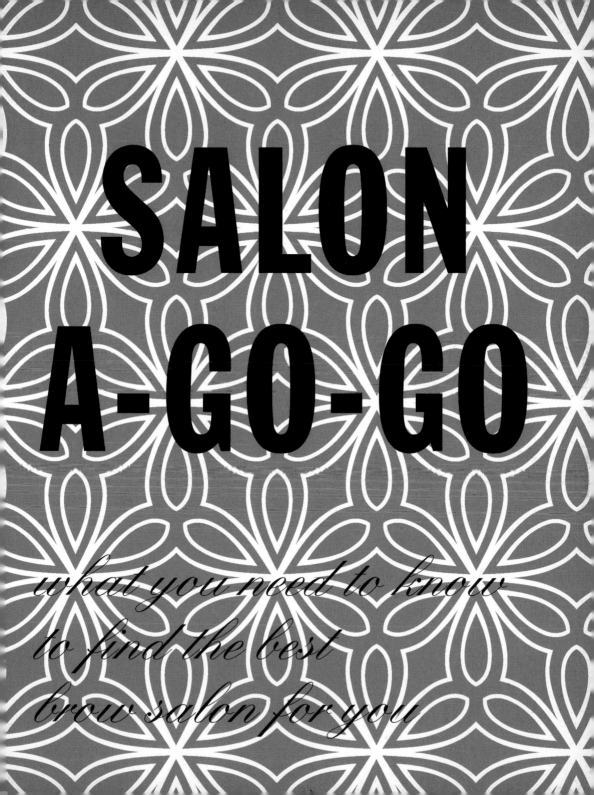

SALON A-GO-GO

what you need to know to find the best brow salon for you

BY NOW YOU SHOULD BE FEELING LIKE A COMPLETE brow expert.

You may even be thinking . . .

Wait. Do I really have to see a professional to get my brows shaped?

If you love your brows, **YES!** You do—seriously.

Not because you need to see a pro but because you *deserve* to see a pro. An aesthetician or professional brow expert is not only trained in the art of brow shaping but also skilled to ensure that the process is fast and virtually pain free and delivers great results. The best aestheticians are up to speed on the latest developments in cosmetics technology and use the highest-quality products available. Yep. The aesthetician does all the work so you get to sit back, relax, and enjoy!

?

AESTHE-WHAT?

Okay. Let's get this out of the way. The word is *aesthetician*.

It's pronounced *es-thi-TIH-shun*. See? Not so hard. It starts out just like the word *aesthetic*. Why? Because an aesthetician is nothing more than a student of aesthetics, a.k.a. a beauty therapist, one trained in the art of enhancing beauty. FYI: Skilled aestheticians come in both the male and female variety.

Here are a few more excellent reasons to get your brows to a salon:

1. It's your face!

2. The skin around your eyes and eyebrows is *very* thin—much thinner than the skin anywhere else on your body.

3. In the brow area, your skin has large nerve trunks close to the surface, which means that whatever happens in this area, you will *really* feel it.

4. A typical brow expert or aesthetician gets months—or years—of professional training and practice before being certified.

> **TRAINING = KNOWLEDGE**
>
> **PRACTICE = SKILL**
>
> **KNOWLEDGE + SKILL = YOUR HAPPY, BEAUTIFUL BROWS**

In chapter 3, we covered the different methods of hair removal on pages 71–72. In this chapter, our focus is on waxing. Waxing is not only the most popular method of removing unwanted brow hair; it's also the most effective (except in a *very* few cases, which we will touch on later in the chapter).

What makes waxing so popular?

It's safe, fast, and relatively inexpensive, *and* it can remove a lot of hair at one time with just one quick tug. It also gives you the longest-lasting results of any method out there because each unwanted hair is pulled out entirely, all the way down to the bulb. No breaks, no stubble, no new hair for weeks!

NOTE TO BROW: For best waxing results, the hairs we want to remove should have at least two weeks of growth.

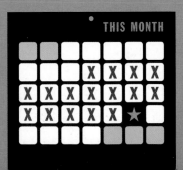

KNOW YOUR
Brow Salon
OPTIONS

Today you can get your brows waxed in a lot of different places. And—**WOW!**—the old adage "You get what you pay for" is so true. Your salon choices for brow waxing fall into three basic categories:

● *High-end spas and salons, specializing in pampering the pants off you before, during, and after your treatment. And it shows in the price. A simple brow shaping can run from $35 to more than $100. Even though you pay a lot, you don't always get a lot of brow-shaping expertise. Most high-end salons focus on facials, massage, haircuts, and other high-ticket treatments, which means that brow shaping isn't an art—it's an afterthought. And the pricey salons that do specialize in brows always require making an appointment in advance. If you have an abundance of time and money or you're looking for a reason to wear a bathrobe out of the house for an hour or two, this is for you.*

● *Brow salons and boutiques, specializing in services for eyebrows and eyes. They are fast and affordable—a typical brow shaping runs about $25—and most welcome walk-ins, so you don't need an appointment. If you have a busy life and want to get the most brow bang for your buck, this is the choice for you. Not only do they specialize in brow and eye services, but they're also better at brow and eye services because that's what they do all day, every day.*✳

● *Nail salons, specializing in quick, inexpensive, backroom, down-and-dirty (emphasis on dirty) services. A nail salon must be really close to where you live or work because, frankly, there's really no other good reason to do that to your brows. If you're a risk-taker on a budget, this is for you.*

THE ADDED BENEFIT

Is this a golden opportunity to mention the many benefits of Benefit Brow Bars and boutiques? You betcha! Benefit Cosmetics opened its first boutique in 1976 and its first brow bar in 2003. Today Benefit has more than five hundred boutiques and brow bars around the world—and more are opening every day. Why? Because the brow experts at Benefit know what they're doing, and all those satisfied customers keep telling their friends and coming back for more BROW-WOW-WOW!

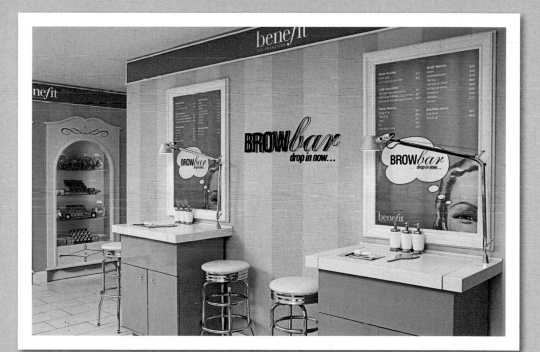

what to look for in a good brow-shaping salon

When choosing a salon or brow boutique for your next brow shaping, it's tempting to base your decision on price or location. Tempting—but risky. (Remember: These are your eyebrows we're talking about—you wear them every day!)

No matter what your budget is, you want a place that offers a clean, comfortable environment with calm, confident aestheticians or brow experts.

When someone is working close to your eyeballs with warm and potentially sharp objects, you want to be sure you're in good (steady) hands. If this is your first time getting a professional brow shaping, be sure to pay special attention to quality, and choose your salon wisely. Like most things in life, you want your first time to be a positive experience—not a mistake that leaves you feeling and/or looking horrified.

Unless you have a personal recommendation from a friend with great brows, you may want to check out in person any salon you are considering. Look around, ask questions, and stay long enough to feel the vibe and see a few happy (or unhappy) customers leaving the salon.

questions to ask before you make an appointment:

● *Who will be doing the work?*

● *What is his/her training?*

● *What tools will be used? Are they used once or sterilized between uses?*

● *What type of wax will be used?*

● *Is the brow wax the same wax you would use on my legs? (If the answer is yes, say no to this brow salon!)*

● *Do you do a brow consultation first?*

If any of the answers leave you feeling uncomfortable, keep looking. There are plenty of great brow places out there.

SALON A-NO-NO

IF YOU SEE ANY OF THESE THINGS, SAY, "JUST BROWSING,"
WAVE POLITELY, AND GET OUT OF THERE:

● EYEBROW STENCILS
(CAN'T REMEMBER WHY? REVIEW THE REASONS ON PAGE 57.)

● A GIANT TUB OF DISGUSTING, WAXY, HONEY-COLORED GOO
WITH A GRIMY LEG-WAXING STICK POKING OUT

● EYEBROWS THAT SCARE YOU—ON THE PROS OR THE CUSTOMERS!

looking for a

threading spot?

If you can't get waxed for medical reasons, or you're simply curious about eyebrow threading, you've got lots of options. Threading, an ancient hair-removal practice, is performed today at all levels of salons, from pricey high-end spas and beauty salons to inexpensive nail salons and kiosks at the mall. (Yes. You read that right! *Kiosks at the mall!*) Not surprisingly, the cost of eyebrow threading varies wildly from $4 to $30—or more when you add in the consultation charge. According to some, threading is *extremely* painful. According to others, it's not painful at all. The experience seems to depend on you (your pain threshold and the amount of hair to be removed) and the skill level of the person doing the threading.

THAT'S WHERE IT GETS INTERESTING.

The training required to become a threading professional is, well, non-existent—there is no formal training. The only equipment needed is a spool of 100-percent-cotton thread. Threading techniques and skills are typically passed on from generation to generation or taught in an old-world apprentice fashion. Watch, learn, try it, be corrected, try again. Like waxing, threading aims to remove the brow hairs at the bulb—but sometimes it breaks them off just under the surface of the skin, which means the hair grows back much faster. Unlike waxing, threading is completely unregulated. So if you do want to give it a try, be sure to find someone you really trust, and get to know her work before you let her near your brows.

A professional brow shaping shouldn't just leave you looking great; it should also leave you feeling great—about the whole experience.

TRUE. YOU COULD JUST GO OUT AND BUY A "PROFESSIONAL BROW-WAXING KIT" TO USE AT HOME. BUT YOU CAN ALSO BUY THE TOOLS TO REWIRE YOUR HOUSE, CHANGE THE OIL IN YOUR CAR, PRUNE YOUR TREES, CUT YOUR OWN HAIR, OR EVEN INJECT YOUR OWN BOTOX. TODAY YOU CAN **DIY ALMOST ANYTHING**—BUT DO YOU REALLY WANT TO? THINK ABOUT IT. YOU DON'T JUST NEED THE TOOLS; YOU NEED THE SKILL TO USE THE TOOLS. THE MONEY YOU THINK YOU'RE SAVING ISN'T WORTH BURNING, BRUTALIZING, OR BOTCHING YOUR BROWS. IF YOU'RE REALLY CRAVING A **DIY ADVENTURE, DO** YOURSELF A BIG FAVOR—LEARN TO CHANGE SOMETHING THAT'S NOT ON YOUR FACE!

Whatever type of brow salon you choose, you should definitely **EDUCATE YOURSELF** about the rules and regulations where you live. Every state (and country) is different. Wherever you are around the globe, be sure that the aesthetician or cosmetologist who will be working on your brows has the proper training and certification. A white coat or sassy smock is not required for great work—but the proper training and paperwork definitely are. It's your assurance that all work performed on your face and brows will be done in a safe and sanitary way.

THE BIG MONEY QUESTION

IF YOU ASK AN AESTHETICIAN JUST ONE QUESTION BEFORE YOU COMMIT, THIS IS THE ONE THAT COUNTS:

WHAT WAS YOUR FAVORITE SUBJECT IN BEAUTY SCHOOL?

WHAT YOU DO WANT TO HEAR:	WHAT YOU DON'T WANT TO HEAR:
BROW SHAPING	BANGS
WAXING	RECESS!
SKIN CARE	BEAUTY SCHOOL?

WHEN TRUSTING YOUR EYEBROWS TO A PRO, YOU DESERVE TO FIND SOMEONE WHO NOT ONLY KNOWS WHAT SHE'S * DOING BUT WHO ALSO LOVES WHAT SHE'S DOING. IT SHOWS IN HER ATTITUDE—AND WILL SHOW IN YOUR BROWS!

*TO KEEP IT SIMPLE, BROW EXPERTS AND AESTHETICIANS WILL BE REFERRED TO IN THE FEMININE. BUT THERE ARE SOME AWESOME MALE BROW EXPERTS OUT THERE, TOO!

questions to ask
BEFORE YOU COMMIT

Are you a licensed aesthetician or cosmetologist (where required)?

Where did you get your training?

What's your approach to brow shaping?

What tools/techniques will you be using?

WAXING? YES.

TWEEZERS? YES.

MICRO MACHETE? NO!

RAZOR? DEFINITELY NOT.

How are your tools sterilized? How often are they sterilized?

NEVER FEEL SHY OR EMBARRASSED about asking these questions! You deserve to know the answers, and any credible professional won't mind answering them. If you get a weird pushback on any of your questions, persist. Clarify the question and ask again. If you're still not satisfied with the answer, graciously excuse yourself.

before the waxing magic happens

Any good, well-trained aesthetician will discuss your medical history with you and offer a consultation *before* whipping out the wax or tweezers. If you aren't offered a personal consultation, you should rethink your salon choice pronto!

LET'S TALK MEDICAL HISTORY

When you sit down with an aesthetician or brow professional, full-frontal disclosure is always the best policy. (Remember: A certified aesthetician is like a beauty therapist, so your medical history and all your brow secrets are protected by the brow doctor–patient privilege.)

If you have any secrets to share, share them now. Let her know if you've had:

● *recent Botox injections*

● *recent brow-lift surgery*

● *recent eye job surgery*

● *recent brow bender (Your brow pro should know the natural thickness of your eyebrows. If you've been overtweezing lately, let her know.)*

Or if:

● *you're on steroids or taking hormone replacement treatment (Either can make your skin more sensitive than usual—not so sensitive that you can't safely get your brows waxed. But do let her know so she can use special care.)*

You may be asked to sign a medical release before any waxing services are performed. This is standard operating procedure in quality salons and protects you as well as the person doing the waxing. Even though a medical release is standard, be sure to read it—and understand it—before you sign it!

THE CONSULTATION

Every great brow shaping starts with great brow mapping.

Remember the brow-shaping basics from chapter 1? Now is when they really matter. Your trained brow expert will apply those basic principles to your face and features as you discuss and map out the best shape for your brows. This is the time to talk about your personal style, what you do for a living, and how much time you typically spend on your makeup, and this is also the time to share any relevant secrets.

AGREE TO THE PLAN

It's smart to go in with an idea of what you want and—just like when getting a haircut—be open to the ideas and expertise offered by the pro. No matter what, you should always feel 100 percent comfortable with the brow plan. It's your face and your decision.

Before any waxing begins, be sure you've agreed on:

1. the start of your brows (your natural Point A)

2. the position of the peak of your arch (your natural Point B)

3. the end of your brows (your natural Point C)

4. the overall shape of your brows

5. the thickness of your brows

Once you've agreed on the mapping of your brows and signed a release, if required, it's time to sit back, relax, and enjoy!

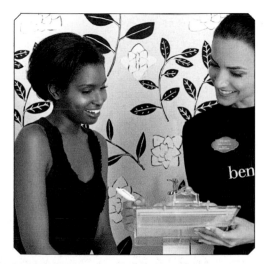
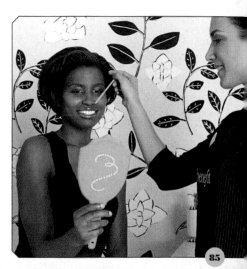

the pro waxing process

First, the aesthetician preps the skin by cleansing it and applying a prewaxing solution to the area to be waxed.

Then she brushes and trims unruly brow hairs.

Next, using a stick or spatula, she applies a thin strip of warm wax in between your brows in the direction in which your hair grows. (The wax should be warm enough to spread easily but not hot enough to burn your skin or feel uncomfortable.)

Next, the aesthetician lays a thin strip of muslin over the wax, smoothing it gently in the direction of your hair growth.

Then a quick tug—like pulling off a Band-Aid—and adios, unwanted hair!

Finally, the aesthetician goes over the area with tweezers, removing any hairs that got away.

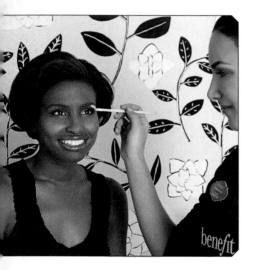 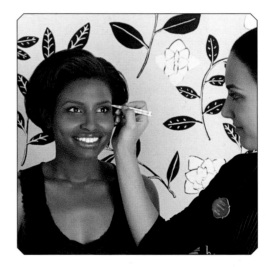

The aesthetician then repeats the same waxing-and-tweezing process above and below the brow, finishing with a wax-removing solution (if needed) and a cooling gel to calm and soothe the skin.

Ouch
MUCH?

SOME PEOPLE WORRY THAT GETTING THEIR BROWS WAXED WILL REALLY HURT.

If you're working with an experienced pro, it doesn't. What hurts more is the fear of the unknown as your brain imagines a world of painful possibilities. Getting waxed is like anything you've never done before—riding a roller coaster, running a half marathon, Internet dating. The big pain comes from not knowing exactly what to expect—or when it will end! Once you've been waxed, you know **THE OUCH FACTOR IS NO BIG DEAL—** and any discomfort you may feel is definitely worth it.

WAXING WARNING

If you've been taking or using any of the following medications within the last thirty days,

DO NOT HAVE YOUR EYEBROWS (OR ANYTHING!) WAXED. SERIOUSLY.

Your skin is *way* too sensitive, and you'll risk losing layers of skin, along with any unwanted hair, which may result in permanent scarring.

- *Retin-A*
- *Renova*
- *Tri-Luma*
- *Differin*

- *any antibiotics*
- *glycolic acid*
- *benzoyl peroxide*
- *any other prescription-strength topical or internal treatment or medication*

If you've taken Accutane within the last six months, pass on the waxing.

Also, do not get your brows waxed if you've had any of the following treatments in the past thirty days:

- *facial peel*
- *laser treatment*

- *microdermabrasion*
- *facial surgery or any other facial procedure or treatment*

Even if you can't get waxed today, you can safely get your brows shaped by a skilled professional using tweezers.

AND JUST TO BE SAFE . . . Don't get waxed if you have a sunburn or if you've recently been drinking alcohol. These cause increased circulation in the surface capillaries, which can make your skin highly sensitive.

THE FORTY-EIGHT-HOUR RULE

After waxing, be sure to wait forty-eight hours before exposing yourself to:

● *the sun*   ● *extreme heat*   ● *any aggressive skin treatments*

Your skin will thank you!

need a quick-release exit strategy?

Are you one of those sweet souls who would rather suffer in silence than maybe even possibly, just a little bit, hurt someone feelings? If you get an uncomfortable feeling from your brow professional—like maybe she has no idea what she's doing—you are free to leave at any point. Really. Permission granted. Do not sacrifice your brows to protect someone else's (imaginary) feelings!

Here are three proven, instant pain-free-for-all exit strategies:

WHAT YOU DO: Casually look at your watch or cell phone, then bolt upright and gasp.

WHAT YOU SAY: "I am *so* sorry, but I'm still on Paris/Tokyo/New York/Sydney time. I'm actually asleep right now. Gotta go!"

WHAT YOU DO: Check your phone for texts, then wince and sigh.

WHAT YOU SAY: "Bummer! My boss/coworker/client/Chihuahua got back early. Apparently I'm late for a previously unscheduled meeting. *Hasta la vista!*"

WHAT YOU DO: Release a huge, fake sneeze, then make your best *uh-oh* face.

WHAT YOU SAY: Oh my. Oh *my*! Terribly sorry. I think I just peed a little in my pants and—I really hope—not in your chair. Pardon me. I'll reschedule.

Regardless of your exit strategy, no one's feelings—or eyebrows—will be hurt.

BROW
Myth
MADNESS

MYTH/FEAR: *Waxing is bad for my skin.*

REALITY: Waxing is actually good for your skin. The warm wax opens the follicles, so it's easier to remove the entire hair right down to the bulb. The best brow waxes contain natural moisturizers that leave your skin feeling smooth and soft.

MYTH/FEAR: *Waxing my brows will make the hairs grow back darker/thicker/faster.*

REALITY: Waxing does not make your brow hairs grow back darker, thicker, or faster. In fact, repeated waxing often causes brow hairs to stop growing. Over time, the follicles get the message and actually stop producing new hair.

MYTH/FEAR: *It's wrong to wax or tweeze above my brows.*

REALITY: Waxing and tweezing *above* the brow is actually the key to creating the perfect arch. (What's wrong is ignoring the unwanted/free-range hairs above your brows!)

raising THE BROW BAR

WITH THE RISING APPRECIATION OF THE GLORIOUS, GROOMED EYEBROW near the end of the twentieth century came the emergence of boutiques and spas specializing in eyebrows. Finally, the well-shaped brow wasn't just an afterthought or an add-on to a facial or other salon treatment—it was the star of the beauty show.

Pricey brow boutiques first appeared in the fashion capitals—Paris, New York, Los Angeles—and initially catered to models, celebrities, and the über brow elite.

But all that changed when Jean and Jane Ford, crazy-for-brows founders of Benefit Cosmetics, opened the first Benefit Brow Bar in 2003—and brought

BROW POWER TO THE PEOPLE!

They listened to their customers and recognized the need for fast, convenient, affordable brow shaping done by a pro. So they made it happen, and they made it fun! (And you don't even need an appointment!) Jean and Jane never considered using stencils (puh-*lease!*) for brow shaping. Instead, they developed their own system for shaping beautiful brows based on the individual features of each customer. Today Benefit has more than five hundred boutiques and brow bars around the world—and more are coming. Benefit didn't invent brow shaping—they just perfected it!✳

Ideally, before leaving the brow bar, you should schedule your next appointment in the next three or four weeks to keep your brows looking their best. But if you're not sure of your schedule weeks ahead of time, no worries. When you walk out of a brow bar after a professional brow shaping, you'll look and feel great and—best of all—you'll be wearing a beautiful brow blueprint (try saying *that* three times fast!) that you can follow at home to keep your brows in shape until your next appointment or drop-in visit.

✳*(Nope. Not an advertisement. Not even an Added Benefit. Just the truth!)*
P.S.: Sometimes the truth is so delicious it makes you want to run out and buy the yummy!

5

MAINTAINING YOUR BROW SANITY

how to keep your eyebrows looking fabulous at home

IN A PERFECT WORLD, THERE WOULD BE
GLOBAL BROW HAPPINESS,

and every woman would have more than enough time and money to get her brows done by a professional every three weeks. But most of us live in the real world, where we have to maintain monthly budgets and busy schedules in addition to our eyebrows. Still, there's no reason for you or your brows to suffer in between salon visits. Here's all you need to know to maintain your beautiful brows at home quickly, safely, and sanely.

FIRST, LET'S TALK ABOUT YOUR TOOLS.

time FOR A trim?

Has it been a while since your last brow salon visit? Are you having trouble taming your brow hairs with a brush, even when using brow gel to style and set them in place? If so, it's probably time for a trim.

HOW DO YOU KNOW FOR SURE? TAKE THE TURTLENECK TEST!

Grab a turtleneck, put it on, and then pull it off in front of a mirror. Do your brows scare you? Do they make you look like someone's Great-Uncle Harry? Time for a trim!

If you don't have a turtleneck handy, just grab a brow brush, lash comb, or an old toothbrush and brush your brow hairs straight up. Are they **HAIRY SCARY?** Do you see any wild ones or leaders of the pack? If so, it's definitely time to get your brows back to the salon. Sure, it's tempting to start trimming your brows at home—but it's not recommended. Trimming your own brows is a lot like cutting your own bangs. Seems like a good idea at the time. Never is.

SNIP. SNIP. OOPS. YIKES!

Even if you're great with scissors, you just don't have the proper perspective to trim your own brows accurately. Invariably, your brows will end up way too short and/or lopsided, and you'll end up feeling like an embarrassed five-year-old who should've known better.

NOTE TO BROW:
Good-bye, Great-Uncle Harry!
Hello, great brow salon!

THE
BEST TOOLS
in the brow shed

The only tools you'll need to keep your brows looking great at home is a mirror (a magnifying one, if you need it), a good pair of tweezers, and a brow brush.

These days you can get all kinds of crazy tweezers—automatic tweezers, tweezers with a built-in LED flashlight, tweezers with a magnifying glass, tweezers with indestructible polymer tips or nonskid gripping panels. But unless you have some very special tweezing needs, stick with the basic models. Why? Because they work the best.

Here are the three most popular types of tweezers:

POINTED SLANT TWEEZERS (also called **NEEDLE-NOSE** or **PRECISION-TIP TWEEZERS**) are typically used for grabbing things under the skin such as ingrown hairs or splinters. These are great if you suffer from ingrown or pesky just-under-the surface dwellers but aren't recommended for everyday maintenance—or for anyone with the caffeine shakes. Use with care! The small, sharp tip makes it harder to connect with your target and easier to pinch your skin by mistake. Ouch!

SLANT TWEEZERS are definitely the most popular choice for tweezing brows and the ones used and recommended by brow experts and makeup artists. The size of the tip makes it easy to pluck individual hairs. And the angle of the tip allows you to hold the tweezers comfortably in your hand so that even if you're a beginner you can tweeze like a pro.

FLAT-TIP TWEEZERS are designed to grab a number of hairs at once, which is exactly what you *don't* want to do. Pass on these for your brows. They're sharp and can easily tear or scratch the delicate skin around your eyes.

quality counts!

The most important factor to consider when shopping for tweezers is quality. Sure, you can pick up cheap tweezers at any drugstore for a few bucks. But **DON'T DO IT.** They just won't work very well. In no time—like immediately—you'll be really frustrated. Tweezing, tweezing, tweezing but not actually gripping or plucking a thing. Do yourself a big favor and buy a pair of quality stainless-steel tweezers. They'll set you back about $20 to $25, *and* they'll be worth every penny.✳ A good pair of tweezers is a precision instrument. So hold on tight! If you drop your tweezers and they land tips-down, you'll need a new pair. All it takes is one crash landing for even the highest-quality tweezers to get out of alignment.

✳ THE ADDED BENEFIT

What's the favorite brand of tweezers among makeup artists, models, and the brow experts at Benefit? Tweezerman. The quality is consistently superior, giving you greater gripping power every time you tweeze. And they come in classic stainless steel or fun colors and supercute prints. No matter what your budget is, the best price-value equation always adds up to Tweezerman!

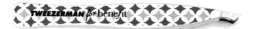

go ahead, be a tweeze!

If you've been dying to tweeze your brows for the past four chapters, **YOU'RE IN LUCK!**
Now you're ready. You've got the right tools, you've learned what goes into shaping
a great brow, *and* you've been to a salon to get your brows shaped by a professional.
Now all you need to keep them looking fabulous is a steady hand and some great light.
Natural light is always best. So if you've got it, use it.

When maintaining your brows at home, your goal is simple: tweeze any new hairs that
grow *outside* the shape created by your brow professional—only the ones that are *obviously* growing wild. You'll want to give your brows a quick examination every few days
to see what's popping up. Tweeze any new free-range brow hairs with confidence. *Do
not* tweeze the new hairs growing in right at or very near your brow line—you know, the
area that actually defines the shape of your brows. This is called the **NO ZONE.** Can you
guess why? Right! When in doubt, don't tweeze a hair right on or near the new growth
line—the No Zone. Make a brow appointment instead. It's so much better to have an
extra hair in your brow for a few days than a hole in your brow for a few weeks.

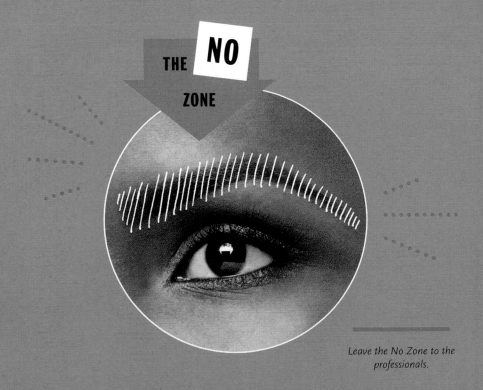

THE **NO** ZONE

*Leave the No Zone to the
professionals.*

STAY OUT
of the No Zone!

The No Zone is the area immediately surrounding your beautiful, well-shaped brow (about a sixteenth to an eighth of an inch beyond the brow). Leave that area to a skilled professional. Once you start tweezing in the No Zone, you begin to mess up the clean lines artfully created by your brow expert. Any at-home brow maintenance should only involve tweezing the wild ones or the hairs that start popping up *outside* the zone.

Keep in mind that eyebrows are not identical twins; they're sisters. So relax. There's no such thing as perfect symmetry in anyone's eyebrows. Just do your best to maintain the new growth outside the lines, and show your brows lots of TLC (tweezer love and care)!

If you're concerned about any crazy brow hairs getting too long in between salon visits, use a brow gel (more on that in chapter 6, on page 118) to tame them until your next brow shaping.

TWEEZING *tips*

Tweezing at home in between visits to your favorite brow pro is a breeze when you follow these tips:

● *Try tweezing right after a hot shower, when your pores are open and it's easier to remove the hairs. (Or use a warm washcloth to open the pores.)*

● *Make sure your tweezer tips are clean and free of any debris that may prevent perfect gripping. Use rubbing alcohol to remove anything sticky or icky that might keep your tips from meeting in perfect harmony.*

● *Tweeze one hair at a time, never groups of hair. (Remember: This is minor maintenance, not major deforestation. Leave that to the pros!)*

● *Always pull hairs out in the same direction in which they grow to avoid breaking.*

● *Tweeze one brow at a time rather than going back and forth between brows.*

● *Once you've got the hair in your tweezers, pull fast! Tweezing only hurts (or makes you sneeze) if you go slowly and drag it out.*

DO YOU SNEEZE WHEN YOU TWEEZE?

IF SO, YOU'RE NOT ALONE, AND YOU'RE NOT WEIRD. (Well, you might be—but not because you sneeze when you tweeze!) What triggers a tweeze-induced sneeze? Just a little nerve-to-brain disconnect. The trigeminal nerve, the largest of the cranial nerves, is responsible for sensation in the face and for certain motor functions such as biting, chewing, and swallowing. One of its three branches, the ophthalmic, monitors what's going on inside your nasal passages and reports back to the brain if it senses anything funky up there. The very same nerve network also monitors sensation in the skin on the eyelids, scalp, and forehead in and around your brows, among other places. Sometimes when tweezing your eyebrows, the nerve gets triggered, and the brain gets the wrong message. Instead of *Scratch my brow!* it senses *Sneeze right now!*

Avoid the miscommunication by pressing on your brow with a finger as you tweeze to short-circuit the nerve, or rub your brow vigorously before tweezing.

GET A GRIP!

NEVER TRY TO TWEEZE A HAIR THAT'S STILL BENEATH THE SURFACE OF THE
SKIN! YOU'LL DAMAGE YOUR SKIN AND GET BACTERIA INTO THE FOLLICLE,
WHICH CAN LEAD TO INFECTION. IF YOU CAN SEE THE HAIR'S PIGMENT UNDER
THE SKIN AND IT BUGS YOU, TRY PUTTING A LITTLE POWDER OR CONCEALER
OVER IT. IF THAT DOESN'T WORK, STEP AWAY FROM THE MIRROR! CHANCES
ARE NO ONE BUT YOU CAN SEE IT. SO JUST FORGET ABOUT IT FOR A DAY OR
TWO, THEN TRY TWEEZING WHEN THE HAIR HAS GROWN THROUGH THE SUR-
FACE AND YOU CAN SAFELY GET A GOOD GRIP.

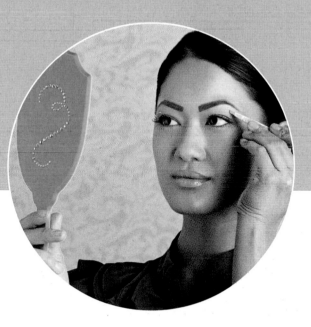

the tweezing afterglow

Depending on the sensitivity of your skin and the thickness of your brow hairs, you may experience a little redness after a big tweeze. To prevent this, finish with a splash of cold water or drench a cotton ball with a soothing astringent such as witch hazel and gently go over the area to cool the skin and close the pores.

IF YOUR SKIN IS RED AND IRRITATED, soak a clean washcloth in a bowl of ice water, then wring it out and press it against the skin. This will close the pores and cause the surface capillaries to contract so the redness diminishes. Or try fresh aloe—the gel inside this succulent is nature's best anti-irritant. Just snap off the end of a leaf and gently dab the irritated area with the gel.

IF THE SKIN IN YOUR BROW AREA IS ITCHY, RED, OR BUMPY, you may need an over-the-counter cortisone cream to cool the heat. But don't worry—the itchiness, redness, or bumpiness won't last long.

don't be a crowd tweezer!

Although a surprising number of people do it, tweezing in public is never a smart plan. You may think you're saving time by finishing your face as you commute to work or rush to a date. And you probably also think you're suddenly magically invisible.

WRONG!

Just because you can't see anyone but yourself in that tiny mirror does not mean that everyone else can't see you! Tweezing in public does *not* make you invisible. It actually makes you *extremely* visible. Unfortunately, you just look like a frazzled fur ball with no personal boundaries and quite possibly no bathroom. Is that really the message you want to send to the world? Didn't think so.

Tweezing in public always raises eyebrows—but never in a good way. **DON'T DO IT. EVER. SERIOUSLY.** Here are some other places where you should never do your tweezing:

BAD PLACES TO TWEEZE

● On an empty elevator (Surprise! What's behind door number 3? You and your unwanted facial hair!)

● In a car or any moving vehicle (That's a moving violation! You're in public—not in your own private vanity case on wheels. P.S.: It will be so embarrassing when you have to explain how you lost an eye.)

● On your bed while the one you love has slipped off to the bathroom or to the kitchen for a—oops! Hi. Back so soon? (It's an image he's not likely to forget and a real mood killer!)

● On public transportation (You're not making up for lost time; you're just making enemies and annoying everyone around you.)

And here are some good ones:

GOOD PLACES TO TWEEZE

● In a bathroom with excellent lighting

● In a bathroom stall with excellent lighting

● In a bathroom with full natural light

● In a bathroom stall with full natural light

● In a bathroom on a plane

● In a bathroom on a train

This is starting to sound like Dr. Seuss, but you get the idea . . .

Eyebrow NO-NOS

DON'T GET CREATIVE.

When you've got tweezers in your hand and your face pressed up to a mirror, it's tempting to explore your creativity. Can I look just a tad more glamorous/artistic/exotic? Can I tweeze a few more years off my face? Can I communicate much more with my brows?

Yes. But don't do it.

An overtweezed, extremely thin brow definitely sends a message. But it's rarely a flattering one. You may think you're telling the world, I'M SUPER GLAM RETRO FABULOUS! But chances are you're actually saying something like, "I've got too much time on my hands." Brow maintenance is not the time to get creative and try to redesign your brow shape. Just follow the lines, and your brows will say everything you want them to.

DON'T DO ANY SOUL-SEARCHING IN YOUR BROWS.

Let's be clear. Brows are important—but not that important. Sure, they can make you look great, but they can't solve your life's problems. If you're placing too much emphasis on your eyebrows, you're at risk of seriously overtweezing.

- *Never search for the meaning of life in your brows.*
- *Never search for your next job/boyfriend/apartment in your brows.*
- *Never search for unconditional love in your brows.*

DON'T TWEEZE UNDER THE INFLUENCE. THAT'S AN AUTOMATIC TUI!

It often starts innocently with a glass of wine or a phone call and then—BAM!—it hits you hard. Suddenly your brows are up against the mirror, and you're anxiously tweezing out of control. It's another tragic case of TUI.

Tweezing under the influence is an underreported cause of eyebrow injury around the world. TUI can be triggered by alcohol or prescription drug use, extreme carbo-loading, casual sugar use, or, worst of all—and most commonly—your crazy female emotions. If you really care about the health and happiness of your brows, just say no to TUI.

NEVER MIX TWEEZERS, EYEBROWS, AND . . .

- cocktails
- fights with boyfriends
- moments of extremely low self-esteem
- insomnia
- homesickness

- wine
- anxiety
- boredom
- sheet cake
- phone calls with your mother

- PMS-induced insanity
- menopause-induced insanity
- breakup-induced insanity
- taxes
- the death of a pet

Please tweeze responsibly—the brow you save may be your own.

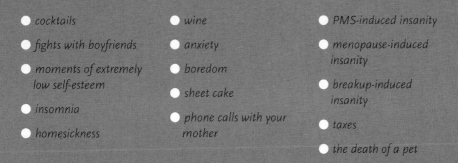

when in doubt, get a brow buddy!

If you don't trust yourself—for whatever reason—when armed with tweezers in front of a mirror, you just might need a Brow Buddy, a trusted friend who understands you and the fine art of brow shaping.

When choosing a Brow Buddy, be sure to consider these things:

- Do we share the same brow values?
- Do we both believe in the power of high-quality tweezers?
- Do we both understand and respect the No Zone?
- Do we vow never to tweeze under the influence?
- Can we stare into each other's eyes without breaking into a sweat or hysterical laughter?

A true Brow Buddy not only offers support and guidance so you can tweeze safely and confidently at home, but she's also there for you 24/7. If you're ever in a brow emergency or about to face one, just call your Brow Buddy's help-line, and she'll talk you down from the tweezing ledge. No judgments, no shame, and no injured eyebrows.

BROW-A-BUNGA!

OH NO. YOU DID IT. YOU WENT COMPLETELY NUTS ON YOUR BROWS and tweezed them into oblivion. Or you thought it would be a good/fast/cheap idea to get your brows waxed by that really nice manicurist in the back room of your nail shop. Oops. Now your brows are lopsided, or scary skinny, or bald and patchy, or completely gone. And now you're totally plucked. **WHAT DO YOU DO?!**

NOTHING.

STAY CALM. Take a breath. It's okay. It's not pretty—but it's also not permanent. Your brow hairs will grow back in a month or two. In the meantime, all you and your brows need is a good, long *stay-away-cation*. Just buy a fabulous pair of oversize sunglasses and leave your brows alone! Don't look. Don't touch. And definitely DO NOT TWEEZE!

(The only reason to even look at your brows during your mandatory *stay-away-cation* would be if you've done so much damage that you need to pencil and/or powder them back in or risk looking like an alien.)

BROW DOUBLE DATE!

IF YOU'RE LOOKING FOR AN EXCITING NEW WAY
TO CONNECT WITH YOUR GUY AND SHARE A BEAUTIFUL EXPERIENCE,
TAKE HIM TO A BROW BAR! MORE AND MORE GUYS ARE
GETTING THEIR BROWS WAXED REGULARLY BY A PRO—
FOR THE SAME REASONS THAT WOMEN ARE
DOING IT: IT'S GOOD FUN AND
GREAT GROOMING!

the guy brow:

YOU AND THE MODERN ART OF MANSCAPING

If you really love your man—boyfriend, husband, brother, dad, roommate, BDF (Best Dude Friend)—then give him a little tweeze. Pull him aside at a quiet, non-embarrassing moment, park him in front of a big mirror, and give him a loving crash course in the art of trimming, tweezing, and taming the furry overgrowth. Most guys will be open to a bit of tasteful manscaping. In ten minutes or less, you'll have a win-win situation. Not only will he look better, but you'll feel better looking at him.

THE BASIC PRINCIPLES FOR GUY BROWS ARE NOT AS STRICT as they are for girl brows. (Remember: Strong, defined brows scream *manly man* in some primitive part of our brain.) But even thick brows need a little TLC (tweezing love and care) to look their best. Your mission is simply to help him tidy the brow area and create a little definition if necessary.

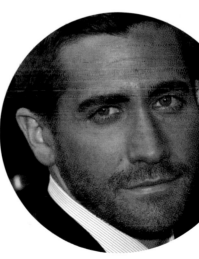

DO:

● *Help him tweeze a healthy—but still manly—path down the middle of a unibrow.*

● *Empower him to pluck any stray, free-range brow hairs that have wandered away from the pack (above and below).*

● *Encourage him to trim any hair longer than about a half inch with brow scissors. (Use your brow brush to comb the brows up and see what needs to go.)*

● *Buy him a great pair of tweezers (and brow scissors if he needs them) as a gift.*

DON'T:

● *Shave anything above the cheekbone.*

● *Do anything drastic or potentially high maintenance. (He's still a guy!)*

6

WOW BROWS

AND

EYE CANDY

*how to take your brows
to the highest level*

makeup!

If you're like most modern women who care about their appearance, you're up to speed when it comes to makeup for your eyes. You have a good understanding of what products are out there:

- eye shadow primer
- under-eye concealer
- mascara

- eye shadow (powder, cream, gel, and stick)
- eyeliner (pencil, powder, and liquid)

- false eyelashes
- eyelash curler

And you know how to use them to look your best.

But even if the contents of your makeup drawer could stock an entire cosmetics counter, you may not be in the know on the **LATEST AND GREATEST** makeup available for enhancing your eyebrows. How could you? The brow game is changing fast.

Back in the day, when your mother's brows knew best, eyebrow makeup options were simple—pencil and powder—*and* they were pretty much just used for brow R&R (rescue and repair). Fast-forward to today.

Wow. Makeup for brows has really improved, expanding into new product areas and benefitting from advanced technology. Now that more people appreciate the importance of beautiful brows, the range of great products designed specifically for brows has become truly inspiring!

Today you can find products that define your eyebrows, adding color, shine, control, and even the illusion of volume. With a little practice and the right tools, you can become your own personal makeup artist, capable of turning your brows into a sexy work of art.

MY BROWS ARE GROOMED,
FULL, AND NATURALLY
FABULOUS.

DO I REALLY NEED PRODUCT
FOR MY EYEBROWS?

THINK OF IT LIKE THIS: IF YOU WANT GREAT HAIR, YOU START WITH A GREAT HAIRCUT. BUT YOU DON'T STOP THERE WHEN YOU REALLY CARE ABOUT HOW YOU LOOK AND WANT YOUR HAIR TO BE AT ITS ABSOLUTE BEST. YOU ADD THE RIGHT PRODUCTS TO ENHANCE YOUR HAIR'S COLOR, DEFINITION, TEXTURE, AND SHINE.

THE SAME IS TRUE FOR YOUR BROWS. (HEY, THEY'RE HAIR, TOO, RIGHT?) EVEN IF YOUR BROWS LOOK FULL AND FOXY AFTER BEING SHAPED, BY ADDING THE RIGHT PRODUCTS YOU CAN GIVE THEM THAT EXTRA WOW POWER—PERFECT FOR SPECIAL EVENINGS OUT OR ANYTIME YOU WANT TO KICK YOUR BEAUTY GAME UP A NOTCH.

FIRST, LET'S TALK ABOUT TOOLS OF THE BEAUTY TRADE.

The eye and brow makeup products you use are only as good as the tools you use to apply them. So be sure to look for quality. They may cost a little more at first, but it's always worth it in the long run. Not only will your brushes last longer, but you'll be able to achieve the results you want every single day without feeling frustrated.

NOTE TO BROW: Frustration causes wincing and frowning—wincing and frowning cause wrinkles! What do wrinkles cause? More frustration! And so on, and so on, and so on. Translation: Buy quality products.

If you spend a little more on tools and products, you're not just investing in the quality of your beauty tool kit—you're investing in the quality of your life!

YOUR *must-have*

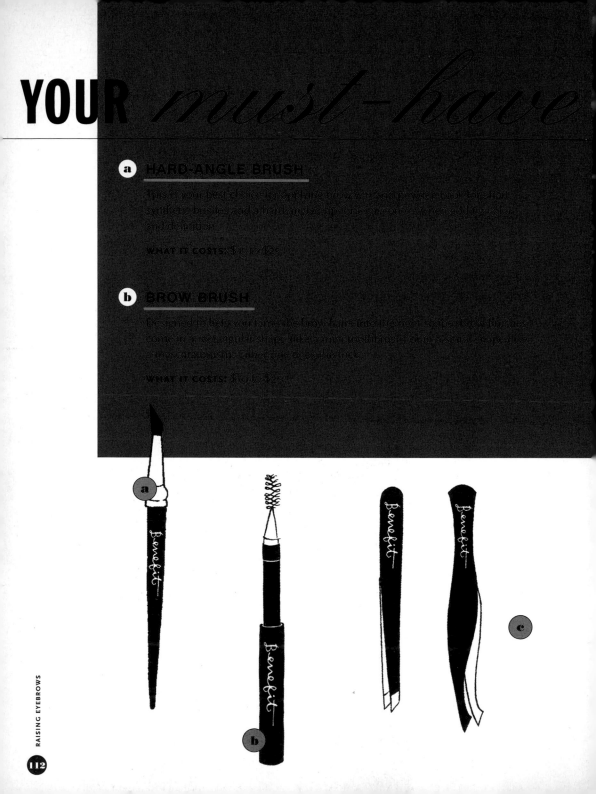

ⓐ HARD-ANGLE BRUSH

This is your best choice for applying brow wax and powder color. Look for short synthetic bristles, and a hard-angled tip for accuracy and ease when adding color and definition.

WHAT IT COSTS: $15 to $25

ⓑ BROW BRUSH

Designed to help you tame the brow hairs into the right shape, brow brushes come in a rectangular shape (like a mini toothbrush) or in a spiral shape (like a mascara brush). Either one does the trick.

WHAT IT COSTS: $10 to $25

BROW TOOLS

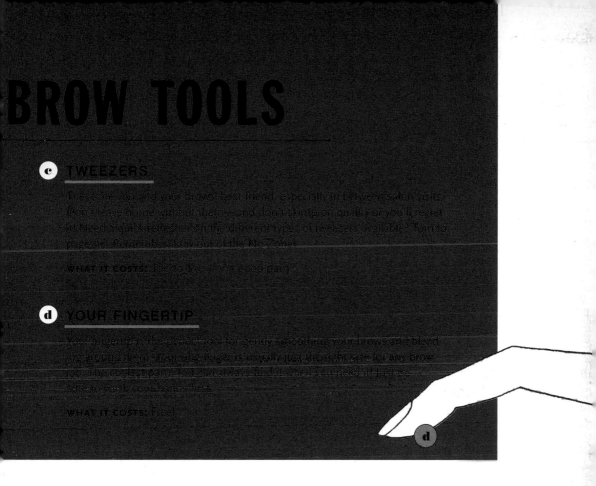

ⓒ TWEEZERS

These are you and your brows' best friend, especially in between salon visits. Don't leave home without them—and don't skimp on quality or you'll regret it. Need a quick refresher on the different types of tweezers available? Turn to page 98. Remember: Stay out of the No-Zone!

WHAT IT COSTS: $10 to $20 for a good pair.

ⓓ YOUR FINGERTIP

Your fingertip is the perfect tool for gently smoothing your brows and blending around them. Your ring finger is usually just the right size for any brow job. The coolest part? You can always find it when you need it. Just be sure to wash your hands first.

WHAT IT COSTS: Free!

ALWAYS KEEP YOUR BRUSHES AND TOOLS CLEAN. A quick, gentle scrub with an antibacterial soap or your shampoo will do the trick. Rinse thoroughly and let them dry flat on a towel. If you leave brushes standing on end when they're wet, water drains down into the base of the brush and breaks down the glue holding them together. (No one needs another breakdown in the bathroom!)

BROW POWER *Products*

Here are all the brow makeup products you'll need to add the most **WOW** to your brow. You can use them individually or in combination—but you do have to use them to make the brow magic happen.

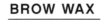

BROW WAX

Add a quick dash of sheer color and a stroke of shine!

WHAT IT DOES: Brow wax adds color to help define your brows, locks unruly hairs into place, and grooms your brows with a touch of shine. It's soft, so it can go on easily with a hard-angle brush, and it comes in dark and light shades or with no color at all.

WHAT YOU DO: Gently drag the side of your hard-angle brush over the wax a few times, then lightly brush over your brows with smooth, long strokes. Always brush in the direction in which your brow hairs grow. Blend the edges with your fingertip. (Be careful not to press so hard that the wax gets on your skin.)

WHAT IT COSTS: About $20 for brow wax alone. The better brands come with brow powder, plus tiny brushes and tweezers, for $30 to $50.

ALWAYS
BRUSH IN THE SAME DIRECTION YOUR BROW HAIRS GROW

BROW POWDER

Enhances definition and creates the illusion of brow perfection!

WHAT IT DOES: Brow powder fills in sparse areas, extends and defines your brow lines, and helps hold your brow hairs in place.

WHAT YOU DO: Gently tap the tip of the hard-angle brush into the powder, then brush over your brows, focusing on areas that need to be filled in, volumized, defined, or extended. Use short, hairlike strokes to create the illusion of hair just where you want it, or follow the edge of your brow line for extra definition. If you need to repair an overtweezing disaster, powder is your go-to girl. It's the best way to make your brows look thicker.

WHAT IT COSTS: About $20 to $30.

BROW WAX AND POWDER

THE ULTIMATE BROW BEAUTY TAG TEAM!

WHILE BROW WAX AND BROW POWDER WORK WELL ON THEIR OWN, THEY WORK EVEN BETTER TOGETHER.* FIRST APPLY THE BROW WAX, WHICH ADDS A HINT OF COLOR AND DEFINITION TO THE BROW HAIRS, THEN ADD THE BROW POWDER TO FILL IN ANY SPARSE AREAS AND ADD VOLUME AND EVEN MORE DEFINITION FOR PERFECT-LOOKING ARCHES. THE WAX ALSO HELPS THE POWDER ADHERE BETTER AND STAY ON LONGER. TRY MIXING THE TWO TOGETHER TO CREATE A CUSTOMIZED BROW COLOR AND DEFINITION. IT'S A WIN-WIN COMBINATION THAT LEAVES WEAK BROWS DOWN FOR THE COUNT!

THE ADDED BENEFIT

Does Benefit offer a killer brow wax and powder combo product? Oh yeah. It's called Brow Zings. Get it? Not to brag, but it's basically the best of the best wax/powder products out there. And it comes in a sleek, sexy, matte black compact with two quality brow brushes and a pair of impossibly cute tiny tweezers. Check it out.

BROW R&R (RESCUE AND REPAIR)

NEED TO FILL IN A TRAGICALLY OVERTWEEZED OR SADLY SHAPED BROW TILL IT GROWS BACK? NO PROBLEM. ALL YOU NEED IS BROW WAX, POWDER, AND A STEADY HAND. START WITH THE WAX, FOLLOWING THE LINE OF YOUR BROW (OR WHAT'S LEFT OF IT), THEN ADD BROW POWDER NOT ONLY OVER THE BROW HAIRS BUT ALSO ALONG THE SKIN RIGHT NEXT TO THE BROW TO EXTEND THE LINE OR THICKEN THE BROW.

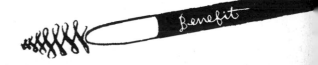

BROW PENCIL

The easiest way to create natural-looking brows on the go!

WHAT IT DOES: A quality brow pencil adds or strengthens color, sharpens and defines the lines of your brows, and fills in any holes or light patches naturally.

WHAT YOU DO: Gently draw the pencil over your brow in short, hairlike strokes, then blend with a brush.

WHAT IT COSTS: About $20 to $30 for the highest quality.

BROW PENCIL TIPS

● QUALITY REALLY COUNTS! THE BEST BROW PENCILS COST A BIT MORE— AND THEY ARE SO WORTH IT! LOOK FOR A SOFT PENCIL THAT GLIDES ON AND LEAVES A NATURAL FINISH (NOT A HARD, HARSH WAXY CRAYON MARK THAT'S IMPOSSIBLE TO BLEND!).

● PAY ATTENTION TO COLOR! TODAY BROW PENCILS COME IN MANY DIFFER-ENT SHADES. TO ACHIEVE THE MOST NATURAL EFFECT, BE SURE TO CHOOSE A COLOR THAT'S CLOSEST TO THE DARKER HAIRS IN YOUR BROWS.

● GO FOR A PENCIL THAT HAS A LITTLE SPIRAL BROW BRUSH ON THE END SO YOU CAN EASILY BLEND AND BRUSH YOUR BROWS INTO PLACE. THAT'S THE KEY TO MAKING PENCILED BROWS LOOK NATURAL.

● KEEP A BROW PENCIL IN YOUR PURSE AT ALL TIMES—AND USE IT! THAT'S THE EASIEST WAY TO BRING UP YOUR BEAUTY GAME INSTANTLY WHEN YOU'RE ON THE MOVE.

BROW GEL

It's all about keeping brows in their place!

WHAT IT DOES: A great brow gel delivers a ONE, TWO, THREE WOW-BROW punch. Brow gel adds a hint of color and shine as it tames your brows into place, and sets them just the way you want them so they'll stay that way.

WHAT YOU DO: Using the mascara-like wand, brush the gel onto your brows in light strokes—always in the direction in which your brow hairs grow. When the gel dries (in seconds), your brows are set—and so are you!

WHAT IT COSTS: About $15 to $20.

FOR MORE
DRAMA
ADD SOME HIGHLIGHTER
ABOVE THE BROWLINE, TOO

BROW HIGHLIGHTER

Want an instant brow lift? (Oh, who doesn't?)

WHAT IT DOES: A brow highlighter is an amazing little secret weapon that adds a glow of light or a shimmer of shine beneath the brow to accentuate its shape. A highlighter opens and brightens the eye area—like an instant brow-lift! Today brow highlighters come in two forms: powder and pencil.

WHAT YOU DO: Apply the pencil or powder just beneath the line of your brow, following the line of the arch. Then blend gently with the tip of your ring finger. When blending, be careful not to rub off the color—a tap and roll motion does the trick. If you want to add even more highbrow drama, add a couple of dots *above* the line of the brow and blend thoroughly.

WHAT IT COSTS: About $20 to $25.

BROW PALETTE

Everything you need to be a brow artist at home or on the go!

WHAT IT DOES: A brow palette contains tinted brow wax, powders, pencil, highlighters, brushes, even tiny tweezers. It helps you add color, definition, shine, and volume, plus it helps tame unruly brow hairs. It also brightens and opens the eye area, comes with a choice of brow powder colors so you can mix the perfect shade for you, and gives you the power to tweeze away any stragglers—any place, anytime.

WHAT YOU DO: Start with a brow wax, then apply a brow powder to add greater definition. (See directions on pages 114–115.) Apply highlighter right under the brow, following the line of the arch. Tweeze any free-range hairs. Look fab!

WHAT IT COSTS: About $35 to $50.

COLOR CORRECTION!

THE BEST BROW PALETTES OFFER MORE THAN ONE COLOR OF BROW POWDER. BUT YOU'RE NOT LIMITED TO CHOOSING ONE SHADE OR ANOTHER. YOU GET TO MIX IT UP! BY BLENDING BOTH COLORS, YOU CAN CREATE THE IDEAL BROW COLOR FOR YOU—DARKER AT NIGHT OR LIGHTER DURING THE DAY. HURRAY!

NOW LET'S PUT IT ALL TOGETHER AND MAKE THE MAGIC HAPPEN.

Of course, before applying any makeup, you always want to start with a fresh, clean, moisturized face. So if you are feeling even a little dirty, now's the time to wash that face!

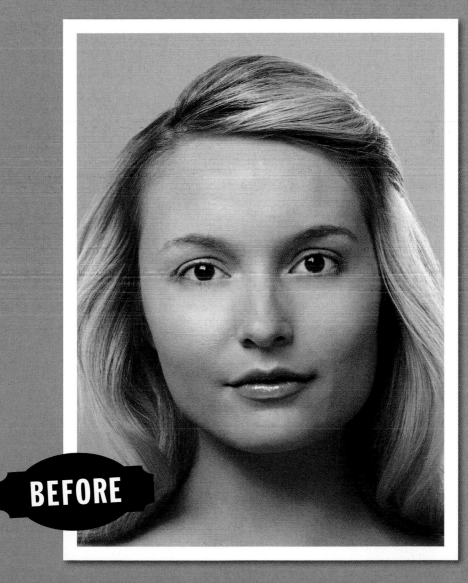

BEFORE

1. Start by applying an eye primer* to the eyelid and under-eye area. This prevents your eye shadow and concealer from creasing and smudging.

* TRY **STAY DON'T STRAY** BY BENEFIT

2. Apply a brightening concealer* to the inner and outer corners of the eye, blending down and around the eye area.

* TRY **ERASE PASTE** BY BENEFIT

3. Apply eye shadow* (both an allover shade and a definer shade).

*TRY **BIG BEAUTIFUL EYES PALETTE** BY BENEFIT

4. Apply eyeliner.*

*TRY **BADGAL LINER WATERPROOF** BY BENEFIT

5. Curl lashes.*

*TRY **PROCURL LASH CURLER** BY TWEEZERMAN FOR BENEFIT

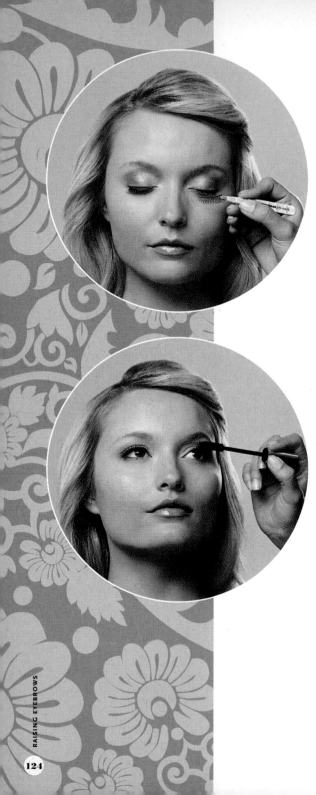

6. Apply false lashes* (if desired).

*TRY **LASH LOVELIES** BY BENEFIT

7. Apply mascara* to upper and lower lashes.

*TRY **BADgal LASH MASCARA** BY BENEFIT

8. Apply brow wax, powder, and/or pencil.✳

✳TRY **BROW ZINGS** BY BENEFIT

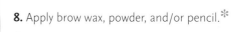

9. Apply brow highlighter.✳

✳TRY **HIGH BROW** BY BENEFIT

10. Finish with brow gel.✳

✳TRY **SPEED BROW** BY BENEFIT

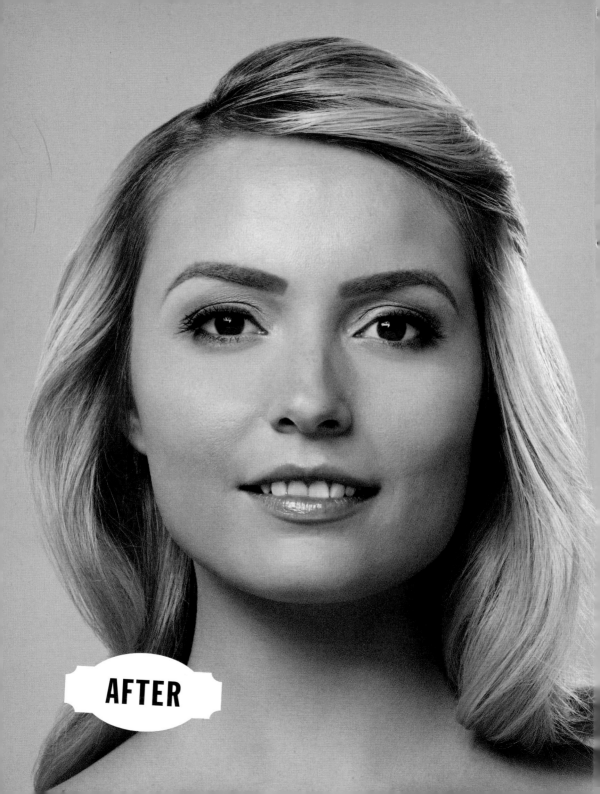

BE A
brow lover
AND AN ACTIVIST
FOR BROW CHANGE!

Take a moment to admire yourself in the mirror. **YOUR BROWS LOOK FABULOUS, AND SO DO YOU!** Now take a bow. You've learned about the many wonders of the eyebrow, passed *Brow History*, and discovered the best brow shape for you—and now you know how to make it happen—at a salon or at home.

CONGRATULATIONS! You have raised your eyebrow awareness and
raised your brows to an art form—but this is just the beginning.

A PARTING GLANCE

Eyebrow styles around the world are as different as the women who wear them. But women everywhere have two things in common—eyebrows and a desire for brow harmony. (Wait. Is that three things?)

YOUR BEAUTIFUL BROWS ARE YOUR TICKET TO GLOBAL GOODWILL. When you raise a well-shaped eyebrow you are speaking a universal language of stylish self-love. Become a brow ambassador and spread the grooming love at home and abroad. As you head out into the world, wear your shapely brows with pride. Use them to connect with more people, ask bolder questions, and make the world a better place.

If you have a friend in need, reach out to her (or him!) with compassionate brow know-how, whether it's your best friend down the street or a Facebook friend on the far side of the world. No brow deserves to go unloved or untended. Now that you've got the knowledge, you can raise eyebrows—and eyebrow consciousness—wherever you go.

MAY THE BROW POWER BE WITH YOU!